MEDICAL TERMINOLOGY from HEAD to TOE

LESLEY BOLTON

Kendall Hunt
publishing company

Kendall Hunt
publishing company
www.kendallhunt.com
Send all inquiries to:
4050 Westmark Drive
Dubuque, IA 52004-1840

ISBN 978-1-4652-9978-9

Printed in the United States of America

Contents

Chapter 1

BREAKING DOWN MEDICAL TERMS, BUILDING UP MEDICAL DEFINITIONS

Medical terminology can be both intimidating and bewildering. It embraces more terms than anyone could likely ever memorize, many of them defying comprehension by their length and complexity. However, you should not despair, for there is a solution. Do not attempt to memorize them all. Instead, master a method of analysis that you can apply to all sorts of new terms that you might encounter, no matter how strange or how lengthy they are. Luckily, the method of analysis is not too difficult. It relies on the fact that many of the medical terms we have today were devised according to a regulated system of rules. If we know the rules, and we apply the system in reverse, we can simply break down troublesome terms into their basic building blocks and then build up the sense of them. Then, distinguishing cardiomalacia, cardiomegaly, and cardiometry becomes a breeze, and confronting a word such as hepatocholangioenterostomy no longer fills us with dread.

You might wonder why terms were devised this way in the first place, if we have to break them down before we can make any sense of them. The answer lies in the history of how medical language and terminology evolved. A detailed knowledge of this is not necessary for our present task, but a summary will highlight some features that will make the task more understandable.

WHERE DID MEDICAL TERMINOLOGY ORIGINATE?

The earliest medical writings of the Western world date back to the ancient Greek world of Hippocrates in the 5th century BCE. While the Greeks did develop a medical terminology of a sort, much of it was based around commonplace language and ideas. The term *catarrh*, for instance, developed in Greek as a combination of the words for "down" and "flow," while the term *thorax* originally described a piece of armor that covered the chest. When Greek medicine was transplanted to Rome in the 1st century CE, Roman writers wanted to compose medical texts in their own language, Latin. Like the Greeks, they had everyday words that served for some technical purposes, but they were hampered by not having an extensive medical language of their own. Their solution was to simply borrow Greek terms and Latinize them, or to take Greek concepts and equate them to Latin ones—for example, they mimicked the Greek idea that "mouth" could be used to mean the opening of any body part and just substituted the Latin word for "mouth" in place of the Greek one.

Latin, along with its Latinized Greek elements, became the dominant medical language throughout Europe, at least in the written tradition, and continued to be so for many centuries. Throughout this time, more and more ordinary Latin and Greek words, but especially Latin, were given a specific medical meaning. Practitioners who could demonstrate mastery of the language might, whether rightly or not, claim some superiority or higher professionalism over those who could not. To be able to read and write Latin, and to some extent Greek, was the hallmark of an educated person. By the 19th century, however, Europeans started writing about medicine in their own languages in place of Latin, although they still incorporated the Latin and Latinized Greek medical terms, with only minor modifications. This era also witnessed a huge rise in "scientific medicine," which, combined with a steady increase in journal publication, encouraged the development of a fresh specialist medical vocabulary. Latin largely provided the basis for a new anatomical nomenclature, while Greek especially became the vehicle for a multitude of systematically-developed compounded terms of the type hepatocholangioenterostomy. In a time when Greek and Latin were still believed to be important elements of a proper education throughout Europe, it made sense to develop new terminology in a language common to all.

Gradually, however, beginning in the 20th century, English started to dominate as the global language for international medical communication, and new terms are now generally based on everyday English, with some national variations. However, the older Greek and Latin terminology remains firmly entrenched in the medical discipline and shows no sign of going away soon.

What do we learn from this history? Well, we learn that a huge percentage of medical terminology is derived from Greek and Latin. It falls basically into three types:

i) Greek and Latin terms that have entered the English language in an anglicized form. Some of them, for example sperm, artery, and nerve were incorporated so long ago that we have ceased to think of them as foreign.

ii) Terms that have entered the English language in their original form. Some terms such as *ganglion* are Greek, but the majority are Latin terms used in anatomy, such as *sacrum*, *vena cava*, and *fossa ovalis*.

iii) Compound terms that were systematically devised. Many utilize Greek base words, as in oligomenorrhea, since the Greek language is particularly suited to forming compounds. However, Latin compounds, such as labiogingival, do occur, as do hybrid terms such as neonatal that mix Latin and Greek elements.

The first type should pose few problems, at least to English speakers. We will spend a little time on the second type, but concentrate mostly on the third type, the compound terms, since these are the most troublesome and the most numerous.

So, on to compound medical terms, and our first objective—breaking them down into plain English that we can understand.

BREAKING DOWN MEDICAL TERMS

Compound medical terms, no matter how long and how complex they are, can be reduced to individual word parts that are the building blocks of terminology. There are just three types of word part: the base, the suffix, and the prefix.

BASE

The base carries the basic meaning and sense of a word. In the term psychiatry, for example, *psych* is the base, with the meaning "mind." It has this same meaning whether we find it in psychology, psychopath, or psychic (a note to students of Greek and Latin, bases in medical terminology generally have only one meaning, perhaps two, not the many variants we see in the ancient languages). Bases always make some sort of sense on their own, since they are modified nouns ("things"), adjectives ("describing" words), or verbs ("doing" words), but their endings are missing. They just need something added to them to make full sense again. Almost all medical terms include a base; those that do not are not derived from Greek and Latin, and do not concern us here. A term can include more than one base, as in psychosomatic, for example, where the bases are *psych* and *som*, meaning "mind" and "body," respectively. Several bases may share the same meaning; *ment*, for instance, also means "mind," but is derived from Latin, whereas *psych* comes from Greek.

SUFFIX

The suffix is added to the end of the base to make meaningful sense. It can be as little as one letter, often a few letters, sometimes more. Just like the bases, almost all medical terms include a suffix, and those that do not are not derived from Greek and Latin, and do not concern us here. The suffix usually makes no sense on its own, but added to the end of the base it forms a complete noun, adjective, or verb. For example, the suffix *osis* makes no sense on its own, but in combination means "abnormal condition of"; when added to the base *psych*, we get *psychosis*, the noun that means "abnormal condition of the mind." Occasionally, a word might have two suffixes following each other. Several suffixes might have the same meaning; *ic* and *al* for example, both mean "pertaining to." These suffixes make adjectives when added to the end of the base, as in *psychic* and *mental*, each meaning "pertaining to the mind."

PREFIX

A prefix can be added to the front of the base. It can be as little as one letter, often a few letters, sometimes more. Not all medical terms include a prefix. The prefix does not make sense on its own; it modifies or adds extra information about the base, telling us how, where, or to what degree something occurs. Prefixes are derived from Greek and Latin adverbs (they tell us "how," "where," or "when"), or prepositions (they tell us "where"). The prefix *endo*, for example, means "within," so *endopsychic* can be understood as "pertaining to within the mind." Occasionally, a word might have two prefixes following each other, but this is not common.

The following table summarizes the prefix, base, and suffix, and their normal use in compound terms:

	prefix	base	suffix
Position in word	beginning	middle	end
Is it essential?	no	yes	yes
More than one?	hardly ever	often	sometimes
Function	adds extra information about the base – often how, where, or to what degree	carries the basic meaning – a modified noun, adjective, or verb with a bit missing	completes the sense of the base – in combination, the suffix and base make a noun, adjective, or verb

There is one more element of the compound term we need to consider. It is not a word part, but an aid to pronunciation—the combining vowel.

COMBINING VOWEL

Consider the word psychotic. We saw above that *psych* is a base that means "mind." We have not met it yet, but *tic* is another suffix that means "pertaining to." Putting the two together would give us psychtic, a rather difficult term to pronounce. Therefore, a combining vowel, "o" in this case, is added to the end of the base to make pronunciation easier. This happens a lot, especially where the base ends with a consonant and the suffix (or another base) starts with a consonant, but in some other odd instances as well. The combining vowel is very often an "o," but sometimes it might be one of the other vowels (a, e, i, u) or y. It adds nothing at all to the meaning. The combining vowel is always considered as added to the end of the base, not the beginning of the suffix.

RECOGNIZING THE WORD PARTS

So, when faced with the compound medical term, what do you do?

i) Identify all the parts. It is a good idea to write the term out, so that you can mark the parts (bracket them, circle them, whatever works for you) as you identify them.

ii) You know that there will be at least one base and a suffix, so find them first. Mark them. Remember, there might be a combining vowel between the base and suffix.

iii) Still have something left over? There probably is not a second suffix, but is there a second base (or even more)? Remember, there might be a combining vowel between the bases. Is there a prefix? Mark everything.

iv) Make sure that nothing is left over. If you have extra letters after marking prefixes, bases, suffixes, and combining vowels, you have gone wrong somewhere and need to start again.

v) When you have identified all the word parts, accounted for any combining vowels, and there is nothing left over, write down the meaning of each individual part. Then, go on to build up the definition.

BUILDING UP MEDICAL DEFINITIONS

So, you have all the word parts identified, and you have their meanings. Now you need to put them together. In many cases, you will have just one base and suffix, perhaps also a prefix. Remember, combining vowels do not have a meaning of their own, and do not alter the meaning of anything.

i) In all cases, BEGIN WITH THE SUFFIX. This is an important point, and it gets the definition off to the right start. It will tell you whether the whole medical term is a noun, an adjective, or a verb.

ii) If you only have a base and a suffix, then the base comes next.

iii) If you have a base, a suffix, and a prefix, then the prefix, since it modifies the base, usually comes next, then the base last of all.

You might need to add in little words, such as "the" and "of," just to make the definition sound right. Here is an example with just a base and a suffix:

	prefix	base	combining vowel	suffix
psychosis		psych "mind"		osis "abnormal condition"
definition order = suffix-base = "abnormal condition of the mind"				

Here, we have a base and a suffix, but also a combining vowel because the base ends with a consonant, and the suffix starts with a consonant:

	prefix	base	combining vowel	suffix
psychotic		psych "mind"	o	tic "pertaining to,"
definition order = suffix-base = "pertaining to the mind"				

This example has a prefix, a base, and a suffix:

	prefix	base	combining vowel	suffix
endopsychic	endo "within"	psych "mind"		ic "pertaining to"
definition order = suffix-prefix-base = "pertaining to within the mind"				

So, the suffix always comes first in the definition, then generally the prefix if there is one, then the base. The combining vowels only help with pronunciation.

What if there is more than one base? For the most part, terms with more than one base follow exactly the same rules. Break the word down into the word parts, build up the definition in the order suffix-prefix(if there is one)-bases. Sometimes, however, the exact relationship between the two bases requires a bit of common sense to be applied. We will meet some terms like this, and we will discuss the different ways of dealing with them as we come across them.

Do not worry if this chapter is a little overwhelming at this stage. It will become a lot clearer when you have learned some prefixes, bases, and suffixes to practice with, but do make sure that you understand what prefixes, bases, and suffixes are, and what they contribute to a medical term, before moving on.

Chapter 2

USING PREFIXES, BASES, AND SUFFIXES TO DESCRIBE THE BODY

Before we go on to look at the body from head to toe, we are going to look at how the body as a whole is described, imagining we are looking at someone standing in front of us, or lying on a hospital bed. This will give us the opportunity to go through how information is presented in the chapters, so that you know exactly what has to be memorized and what has to be understood.

Most of the new prefixes and suffixes will be introduced in the first half of the book. These will be in tables at the beginning of the chapters. You must memorize all of the prefixes and suffixes, and all of their meanings. You will use them over and over again, not just in the chapter they are introduced.

Whenever a new term is introduced, try to think of an everyday term that might help you remember the meaning. Write it in the margin of the page.

Here are the prefixes and suffixes to learn for this chapter.

PREFIXES

Remember, the prefix is added to the front of the base. It modifies or adds extra information about the base, telling us how, where, or to what degree something happens. Not all terms have a prefix. In the tables, the prefixes (italicized) are followed by a hyphen, because they go before another word part, almost always a base. Some prefixes have more than one meaning; you must learn all the prefixes and all of their meanings.

1. *ambi-, ambo-*	both
2. *apo-*	away
3. *contra-*	opposite, against
4. *ecto-*	outside, outer
5. *endo-*	inside, inner
6. *inter-*	between
7. *intra-*	within
8. *meso-*	middle
9. *sub-*	below, underneath
10. *super-*	upper, above, beyond
11. *trans-*	across, through

Because we are looking at ways of describing the body, a lot of these prefixes tell us where something occurs. *ambi-* and *ambo-* are just alternative forms of the same prefix.

SUFFIXES

Remember, the suffix is added to the end of the base to make meaningful sense. The base and suffix together form a complete noun, adjective, or verb. All of the compound terms we will be looking at have a suffix. In the tables, the suffixes are preceded by a hyphen, because they go after another word part, almost always a base. Some suffixes have more than one meaning; you must learn all the suffixes and all of their meanings.

1. -ad	toward
2. -an	pertaining to
3. -al	pertaining to
4. -ary	pertaining to
5. -ial	pertaining to
6. -ic	pertaining to
7. -ion	action, condition, act of
8. -ior	pertaining to
9. -ous	pertaining to, like, full of, having
10. -tic	pertaining to
11. -verse	to turn, to travel, turned

You will find that a lot of suffixes mean "pertaining to." They form an adjective ("describing" word) when combined with a base. A suffix such as -ion forms a noun ("thing") when combined with a base. The suffix -verse is a little unusual, since it is actually a base (VERS-) and suffix (-e) combined, but we will treat it for the moment as if it is a regular suffix. It can form a verb or verb part ("doing" word) when combined with a base, but can also form a noun or an adjective. The suffix -e does not have a meaning of its own.

BASES

Every chapter introduces some new bases. The bases (capitalized) are followed by a hyphen, because they go before another word part, either another base or a suffix. Each base is then followed by a definition, or several related definitions. Then, below the entry, are one or more examples of its use in a compound term, showing how it can combine with other word parts, and sometimes some further explanation or comments. You do not need to memorize the compound terms; they are here as examples. If you learn all of your prefixes, bases, and suffixes, you will never need to memorize the meaning of compound terms. However, do make sure that you understand what the individual word parts are, and how they are combined. Some bases have two meanings that are entirely different—these are marked as (i) and (ii) in the definition line; you must learn all the bases and all of their meanings.

1. **VENTR—front, abdomen, belly**

    ventral (VENTR-al) – pertaining to the front

    ventrad (VENTR-ad) – toward the front

2. **DORS—back**

    mesodorsal (*meso*-DORS-al) – pertaining to the middle of the back

    dorsoventral (DORS-O-VENTR-al) – pertaining to the front and back

    dorsad (DORS-ad) – toward the back

The front side of the body is the ventral surface or ventral section. The back side of the body is the dorsal surface or dorsal section. Inside the body, there is the ventral cavity at the front of the body, and the dorsal cavity at the back. If you lie on your back, you are in a dorsal position. If you move toward the front, you are moving in a ventrad direction, and if you move toward the back, you are moving in a dorsad direction.

3. **ANTER—front, before**

    anterior (ANTER-ior) – pertaining to the front

4. **POSTER—back, behind**

    posterior (POSTER-ior) – pertaining to the back

5. **FRONT—front, forehead**

    frontal (FRONT-al) – pertaining to the front

Anterior and posterior also relate to the front and back of the body, just like ventral and dorsal, but they also have a special meaning. This is because they are originally Latin comparative adjectives that mean something like "nearer" and "further." Therefore, if a structure is anterior, it means it is nearer to the front, while a posterior structure is further to the back. Lots of things in the body occur in pairs, so you might find an anterior and posterior pair, like the anterior and posterior cruciate ligaments in the knee. There is also a very particular use of the term frontal; the frontal bone of the skull, which forms the forehead and top of the skull.

6. **LATER—side**

    contralateral (*contra*-LATER-al) – pertaining to the opposite side

    ambilateral (*ambi*-LATER-al) – pertaining to both sides

7. **MEDI—middle, midline**

    median (MEDI-an) – pertaining to the middle

    mediad (MEDI-ad) – toward the middle

8. **MES—middle, midline**

   mesal (MES-al) – pertaining to the middle

   mesial (MES-I-al) – pertaining to the middle

Both MES- and MEDI- have the same meaning; they are just derived from Greek and Latin forms, respectively. If you are interested as to which terms have come to us from Greek and which from Latin, any good medical dictionary will tell you, but you do not need to know for our purposes. Note that the combining vowel in mesial is "i."

9. **CENTR—center, mid-point**

   apocentric (*apo*-CENTR-ic) – pertaining to away from the center

10. **DEXTR—right, right-handed**

    dextrad (DEXTR-ad) – toward the right

11. **SINISTR—left, left-handed**

    sinistrad (SINISTR-ad) – toward the left

12. **LAEV—left, left-handed**
    LEV—left, left-handed

    levoversion (LEV-O-VERS-ion) – action of turning to the left

LAEV- is the British spelling of LEV-; you will probably come across both forms. Both bases LEV- and SINISTR- indicate the left. Like MES- and MEDI- above, they are derived from Greek and Latin forms, respectively. The term levoversion has two bases, LEV- and VERS-; remember we said that many compound terms have more than one base. The combining vowel "o" is added to the base LEV- to make pronunciation easier, since LEV- ends with a consonant and VERS- begins with a consonant. We will often see the combining vowel appear between bases, and between bases and suffixes; remember, it is very often the letter "o."

13. **SUPER—above, in the top part of**

    superior (SUPER-ior) – pertaining to above

14. **INFER—below, in the bottom part of**

    inferior (INFER-ior) – pertaining to below

Like anterior and posterior, superior and inferior are comparative Latin adjectives, and they can mean something like "higher" and "lower." Therefore, if a structure is superior, it is closer to the higher up part of something, while an inferior structure is closer to the lower down part of something. Again, you can find things in the body in pairs, such as the superior and inferior venae cavae, the veins that carry blood into the heart.

15. CEPHAL—head

cephalic (CEPHAL-ic) – pertaining to the head

intracephalic (*intra*-CEPHAL-ic) – pertaining to within the head

cephalad (CEPHAL-ad) – toward the head

caudocephalad (CAUD-O-CEPHAL-ad) – toward the head from the tail

16. CAUD—tail (in humans, the tail bone or coccyx)

caudal (CAUD-al) – pertaining to the tail

caudad (CAUD-ad) – toward the tail

cephalocaudad (CEPHAL-O-CAUD-ad) – toward the tail from the head

Both caudocephalad and cephalocaudad include two bases; in each case, the combining vowel "o" is added to the first of the two bases to make pronunciation easier.

17. PROXIM—near to, near a point of attachment, near the beginning of a structure

proximal (PROXIM-al) – pertaining to near to the point of attachment

18. DIST—away from, away from a point of attachment, away from the beginning of a structure

distal (DIST-al) – pertaining to away from the point of attachment

The terms proximal and distal are often used about limbs and bones, and we can usually think in terms of closer to, or further away from, the trunk of the body. The most distal parts of the arms and legs are the finger- and toe-tips; their most proximal parts are where they meet the shoulders and hips. The distal end of the shin bone is at the ankle joint, while its proximal end is at the knee joint.

19. INTERN—inside

internal (INTERN-al) – pertaining to the inside

20. EXTERN—outside

external (EXTERN-al) – pertaining to the outside

21. FACI—face, surface
-FICI—face, surface

facial (FACI-al) – pertaining to the face

superficial (*super*-FICI-al) – pertaining to the upper surface

Here, there are alternative base forms, FACI- and -FICI-, both with the same meanings; the form -FICI- only occurs in the middle of a term, never at the beginning. Note also that we are using the prefix *super-* here, and not the base SUPER-. The prefix is modifying the base, telling us something extra about it; in this case, it tells us where something occurs—the upper part of the surface. Structures that are on or near the surface of the body are termed superficial or external; structures that are below or inside the body are termed deep or internal.

22. PARIET—wall (usually, of a body cavity)

parietal (PARIET-al) – pertaining to a cavity wall

interparietal (*inter*-PARIET-al) – pertaining to between cavity walls

intraparietal (*intra*-PARIET-al) – pertaining to within cavity walls

transparietal (*trans*-PARIET-al) – pertaining to across cavity walls

Remembering the difference between the prefixes *inter-* and *intra-* can be tricky. Think of everyday words that might help you distinguish them. Write them in the margin of the page. There is also a very particular use of the term parietal; the parietal bones of the skull. These two bones form the upper sides and back of the skull; they each have four "walls" (edges), and together they "house" a large part of the brain.

23. AX—axis, central line

axial (AX-ial) – pertaining to a central line

subaxial (*sub*-AX-ial) – pertaining to below the central line (of the body)

A lot of the bases we have looked at here relate to dividing the body into two parts: front and back, top and bottom, and left and right. Medical terminology often talks about the body as if imaginary planes, like flat sheets of glass, pass through the body to create these parts. If you think of these planes occupying the axial lines that go through the central lines of the body, there are three positions they can occupy, one horizontal plane and two vertical planes. These planes got their special names, transverse, coronal, and sagittal, using the next three bases.

24. VERS—travel, turn
VERT—travel, turn

transverse (*trans*-VERS-e/*trans*-verse) – travel across

version (VERS-ion) – the action of turning

If our imaginary plane passes through the central line of the body horizontally at the abdomen, it cuts the body into the superior and inferior sections. The imaginary plane is termed the transverse plane. Sometimes, bases (and prefixes and suffixes) can have alternate spellings, depending on what other word parts they combine with, as here with VERS- and VERT-. Memorize all the forms that are listed. We saw above that the base VERS- and the suffix -e create the term -verse, which is often considered to be a suffix in its own right.

25. CORON—crown, like a crown

coronal (CORON-al) – pertaining to like a crown

coronary (CORON-ary) – pertaining to like a crown

26. SAGITT—arrow

sagittal (SAGITT-al) – pertaining to an arrow

Both the coronal plane and sagittal plane got their names in a more complicated way than the transverse plane. The form CORON- has come to mean something circular like a crown you wear on your head, or anything that encircles something else. Some of the bones of the human skull are held together by fibrous bands known as sutures; one of these is the coronal suture. It travels approximately from between eye and ear on one side, going across the top of the head, down to between eye and ear on the other side, in roughly a circular route (probably how you would wear a tiara, rather than a crown). If our imaginary plane passes through the central line of the body, lined up in exactly the same direction as the coronal suture, it cuts the body into the anterior and posterior (or, ventral and dorsal) sections. The imaginary plane is termed the coronal plane. Anything that is coronary acts like a crown in that it encircles something; so, coronary nerves, blood vessels, and ligaments surround other anatomical structures.

The sagittal plane also gets its name from a suture in the skull. The sagittal suture joins the parietal bones (see above), traveling perpendicular to the coronal suture and from the front of the skull to the back. Assuming that you were facing your enemy in olden times, and not running away, if you were shot by an arrow, it pierced you from front to back; this is how sagittal has come to have a special meaning of "pertaining to the direction front to back." If our imaginary plane passes through the central line of the body, lined up in exactly the same direction as the sagittal suture, it cuts the body into the left and right sections. The imaginary plane is termed the sagittal plane.

27. MORPH—form, shape

morphic (MORPH-ic) – pertaining to shape

morphous (MORPH-ous) – pertaining to shape

morphotic (MORPH-O-tic) – pertaining to shape

In morphotic, the combining vowel "o" is added to the base to make pronunciation easier, since both base and suffix begin with a consonant.

28. DERM—skin, layer
DERMAT—skin, layer

endodermic (*endo*-DERM-ic) – pertaining to an inside layer

mesodermic (*meso*-DERM-ic) – pertaining to a middle layer

ectodermic (*ecto*-DERM-ic) – pertaining to an outside layer

These three terms can be applied to the layers of tissues in the developing embryo. According to one classification system (now somewhat discredited), a predominance of any one tissue affects the physique of an individual. Thus, those who have a predominance of endodermic tissue are described as endomorphic (*endo*-MORPH-ic), and are physically rounded, those with a predominance of ectodermic tissue are described as ectomorphic (*ecto*-MORPH-ic) and are physically slender, while those with a predominance of mesodermic tissue are described as mesomorphic (*meso*-MORPH-ic), and are physically well proportioned.

Finally, two bases that relate to the body as a whole (or, the main body of a structure):

29. SOM—body
SOMAT—body

somal (SOM-al) – pertaining to the body

somatic (SOMAT-ic) – pertaining to the body

30. CORP—body
CORPOR—body
CORPUS—body

corporal (CORPOR-al) – pertaining to the body

SOME THINGS TO NOTE

Do not worry that there are several ways of saying the same thing. There are lots of suffixes, for example, that mean "pertaining to." Just accept that this is how it is. In addition, we have seen that there are sometimes terms derived from both Greek and Latin that mean pretty much the same. Again, just accept it, and learn both forms.

We said in the last chapter that terms with more than one base can sometimes be challenging to deal with. This chapter introduced four compound terms that include two bases—dorsoventral, levoversion, caudocephalad, and cephalocaudad. All have the format BASE-BASE-suffix, with a combining vowel between the bases. How do we deal with them? After breaking the term into its component parts, begin, as always, with the suffix and the base nearest it;

we will call this the ultimate base (i.e., the last), we will call the one before it the penultimate (i.e., the next to last). So, beginning with the suffix and the ultimate base:

dorsoventral (DORS-O-VENTR-al) – pertaining to the front …
levoversion (LEV-O-VERS-ion) – action of turning …
caudocephalad (CAUD-O-CEPHAL-ad) – toward the head …
cephalocaudad (CEPHAL-O-CAUD-ad) – toward the tail …

We can ignore the combining vowel because it adds nothing to the sense. The problem now is how the penultimate base relates to the rest of the term. Often you will find that the two bases can be linked with the word "and." This works perfectly for dorsoventral:

dorsoventral (DORS-O-VENTR-al) – pertaining to the front and back

The suffix -al is actually completing the sense of both bases. Sometimes, however, "and" just will not work. In the term levoversion, it obviously makes no sense at all. In caudocephalad and cephalocaudad, it might initially seem plausible, but when we think about it, we cannot be moving in opposite directions at the same time. In these cases, the suffix is only completing the sense of the ultimate base; the penultimate base is actually giving us more information about the ultimate base. We just have to apply a bit of common sense and think about what is the most likely meaning:

levoversion (LEV-O-VERS-ion) – action of turning to the left
caudocephalad (CAUD-O-CEPHAL-ad) – toward the head from the tail
cephalocaudad (CEPHAL-O-CAUD-ad) – toward the tail from the head

Do not worry, this becomes much easier with practice and you will start to see patterns of certain types of compound terms that will help you figure this out. The most important thing for the moment is to make sure you memorize all of the prefixes, bases, and suffixes, including any variable spellings, and all of their possible meanings, and to fully understand how the individual word parts are combined in the examples.

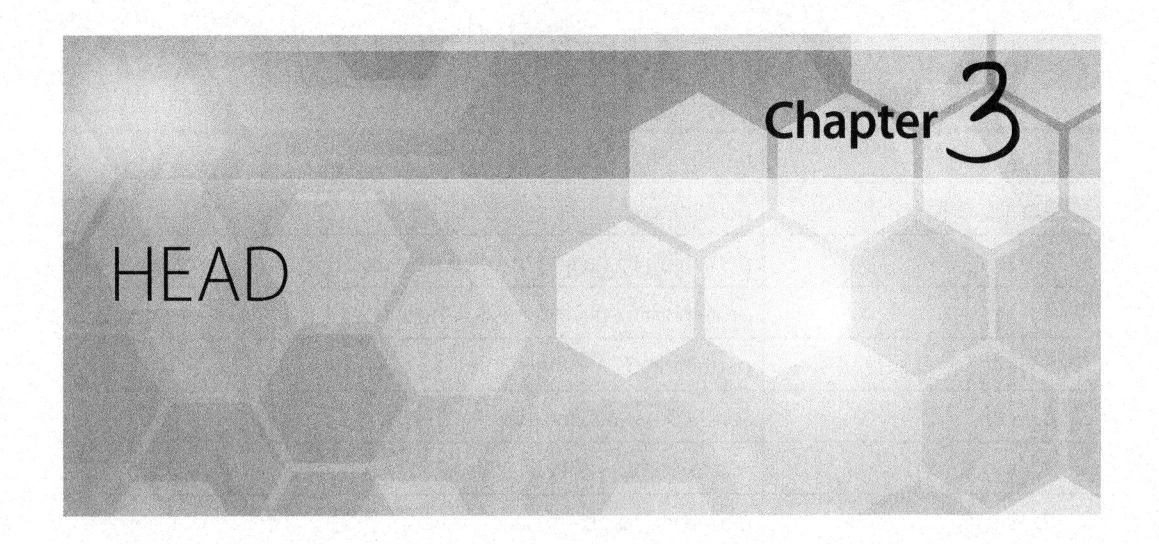

Now we will begin our journey through the body, beginning with the head. As always, whenever a new term is introduced, try to think of an everyday term that might help you remember the meaning. Write it in the margin of the page.

PREFIXES

1. *a-*	without, not, non-
2. *anti-*	against, opposite
3. *circum-*	around
4. *de-*	down, downward, away from, from, without, out of
5. *dys-*	bad, painful, difficult, abnormal
6. *en-*	in, inward
7. *epi-*	upon, on the surface
8. *eu-*	good, well, normal
9. *hyper-*	over, above, more than normal
10. *hypo-*	below, deficient, less than normal
11. *peri-*	around, near

SUFFIXES

1. -al, -eal, -ial	pertaining to
2. -alis, -aris	pertaining to
3. -ar	pertaining to, having the character of
4. -ate	pertaining to, having, having the shape of, to (...)
5. -etic	pertaining to
6. -ety	condition, state, quality
7. -ia	condition of, quality of, state of, act of
8. -ile	pertaining to, able to
9. -ity	condition, state, quality
10. -ive	pertaining to, tending to
11. -oid	resembling, shaped, like, shaped like
12. -orium	place for
13. -osis	process of, condition of, abnormal condition of
14. -sia, -sis,	process of, condition of, act of
15. -ure	result of, act of
16. -y	condition of, quality of, state of, act of

Note how suffixes can have alternative forms; the suffixes -al, -eal, and -ial are just different forms of the same suffix. Likewise, the suffixes -sia and -sis both have the same origin and mean the same; the suffix -osis is also related to them. The form -aris is more common than -alis after bases that have the letter "l" close to the end, but, in most cases, there are no simple rules to explain why one form of the suffix is preferred over another in any particular term. You need to learn the alternative forms.

The bases introduced in each chapter are presented according to the body part. They are not organized according to body systems, so you get a mix of terms relating to bones, organs, diseases, and more. Other general bases are also introduced, so that we can make more compound terms.

Sometimes, you have to use a bit of common sense to fully understand a compound term, even after you have broken it down and then built up the individual parts. A dictionary type definition is given after some terms; you do not have to memorize them, but make sure that you understand how the basic meaning of the compound term has been extended to suit a specific circumstance.

BASES

1. **CRANI—cranium (skull or, more correctly, the part of the skull that does not include the jawbone)**

    craniate (CRANI-ate) – pertaining to the cranium

    circumcranial (*circum*-CRANI-al) – pertaining to around the cranium

    epicranial (*epi*-CRANI-al) – pertaining to on the surface of the cranium

The skull is made up of the cranium and the mandible (jawbone).

2. **TEMPOR—(i) temple (side of the head, behind and above the ear): (ii) time**

    temporal (TEMPOR-al) – pertaining to the temple, pertaining to time

    temporalis (TEMPOR-alis) – pertaining to the temple, pertaining to time

    temporoparietal (TEMPOR-O-PARIET-al) – pertaining to the parietal and temporal bones or regions

The base TEMPOR- can mean both temple and time. You have to decide from context which is most suitable; in medical language, it is most likely to be the temple. There is also a very particular use of the term temporal; the temporal bones, the two bones that form the lower sides of the cranium, behind and above the ears. We came across the frontal and parietal cranial bones (CRANI-al—relating to the cranium) in Chapter 2, where their medical terms made specific uses of the bases FRONT- and PARIET-. Remember, these are very specific uses and not the only occasions where you might come across these bases.

3. **OCCIPIT—occiput (back of the head)**

    occipital (OCCIPIT-al) – pertaining to the occiput

    perioccipital (*peri*-OCCIPIT-al) – pertaining to around the occiput

    occipitotemporal (OCCIPIT-O-TEMPOR-al) – pertaining to the temporal and occipital bones or regions

Again, there is a very particular use of the term occipital; the occipital bone, the large bone at the back of the cranium that extends to the underside.

4. **SPHEN—wedge**

   sphenoid (SPHEN-oid) – shaped like a wedge

   sphenocephalic (SPHEN-O-CEPHAL-ic) – pertaining to a head that is wedge shaped

   sphenofrontal (SPHEN-O-FRONT-al) – pertaining to the frontal and sphenoid bones or regions

Yet again, a very particular use of the term sphenoid; the sphenoid bone is a large bone at the base and sides of the cranium, which also forms part of the eye sockets. Is it wedge shaped? Depends on how you visualize a wedge; a regular trapezium is probably the closest technical description of the shape, but it also looks a little like a butterfly. On each side of the sphenoid, a pair of bony plates, the medial and lateral pterygoid plates, project downward.

5. **PTER—wing**
   PTERYG—wing

   pterous (PTER-ous) – having wings

   pterygoid (PTERYG-oid) – resembling a wing

   apterygial (*a*-PTERYG-ial) – pertaining to without wings

The following two bases also relate to bones of the cranium, or their associated regions. You will probably only ever come across these bases in compound terms relating to the head and these bones.

6. **ETHM—sieve**

   ethmoid (ETHM-oid) – resembling a sieve

The ethmoid bone, located behind the nose, has a lot of open spaces in it, just like a sieve.

7. **ZYGOMAT—yoke**

   zygomatic (ZYGOMAT-ic) – pertaining to a yoke

The zygomatic bone, the cheek bone that extends to the edge of the eyes socket, is shaped somewhat like the yoke you might place on oxen ploughing land. The base ZYG-, which gives us the term zygote, also means yoke.

8. **SQUAM—scale**

   squamous (SQUAM-ous) – having scales

While in zoology this base does have the meaning "scale," in medical terminology its sense has been extended to "scale shaped" or "scalelike," so the term squama can mean both a thin plate of bone (i.e., a scalelike piece of bone) and a cell that is shaped like a thin scale. The frontal, occipital, and temporal bones all have squamous regions:

SQUAM—scalelike bone, scalelike cell, squama

squamous (SQUAM-ous) – having scalelike bone, having scalelike cells

squamofrontal (SQUAM-O-FRONT-al) – pertaining to the frontal bone squama

squamotemporal (SQUAM-O-TEMPOR-al) – pertaining to the temporal bone squama

9. LAMBD—Greek letter lambda (λ)

lamdoid (LAMBD-oid) – shaped like the Greek letter lambda

The lambdoid suture (sutures are fibrous band between cranial bones), between the occipital and parietal bones, is shaped like the Greek letter lambda, sort of an upside down Y.

10. SIGM—Greek letter sigma (ς)

sigmoid (SIGM-oid) – shaped like the Greek letter sigma

Another base coming from the Greek alphabet, anything that is sigmoid is shaped like the Greek letter sigma, that is "S shaped." The sigmoid sinus (a sinus is a hollow channel) of the cranium travels through an S-shaped channel.

11. CAV—hollow space

cavity (CAV-ity) – condition of a hollow space

Notice how the suffix -ity forms a noun when added to a base. The cranial cavity, inside the cranium, contains the brain and related structures.

12. CEREBR—cerebrum (largest part of the brain)

cerebral (CEREBR-al) – pertaining to the cerebrum

intracerebral (*intra*-CEREBR-al) – pertaining to within the cerebrum

13. CEREBELL—cerebellum (the posterior part of the brain)

cerebellar (CEREBELL-ar) – pertaining to the cerebellum

14. ENCEPHAL—brain

encephalic (ENCEPHAL-ic) – pertaining to the brain

encephaloid (ENCEPHAL-oid) – resembling the brain or brain substance

periencephalic (*peri*-ENCEPHAL-ic) – pertaining to around the brain

We met the base CEPHAL-, "head," in Chapter 2. ENCEPHAL- is actually a compound of CEPHAL- with the prefix *en*- meaning "in," but it has also become used as a base in its own right.

15. LOB—lobe

lobate (LOB-ate) – having lobes

sublobar (*sub*-LOB-ar) – pertaining to below a lobe

A lobe is a division or extension of an organ or part.

16. FISS—split, splitting

fissure (FISS-ure) – the result of splitting

fissile (FISS-ile) – able to be split

Notice how the suffix -ure forms a noun when added to a base. A fissure is a deep slit or cleft; in the brain, a fissure divides the cerebrum into left and right lobes.

17. THALAM—chamber, thalamus

thalamic (THALAM-ic) – pertaining to the thalamus

hypothalamic (*hypo*-THALAM-ic) – pertaining to below the thalamus

The base THALAM- comes from the Greek word for a bedroom, especially a bridal chamber. The great physician Galen compared the layout of a Greek house to the layout of the brain; since the bridal chamber played a central and crucial role in the ancient household, he gave the name thalamus to the structure he saw fulfilling a central and crucial role in the functioning of the brain. The hypothalamus is located below the thalamus.

18. MENING—membrane, meninges

meningeal (MENING-eal) – pertaining to the meninges

submeningeal (*sub*-MENING-eal) – pertaining to below the meninges

The base MENING- is used almost exclusively about the membrane layers that surround the brain and spinal cord, the meninges.

19. ARACHN—spider, spiderweb

arachnoid (ARACHN-oid) – resembling a spiderweb

One of the meninges is the arachnoid, a delicate spiderweb-like layer. Beneath the arachnoid is the subarachnoid (*sub*-ARACHN-oid) space. In Greek mythology, Arachne was a mortal woman who boasted that she could weave better than anyone, even the immortals, prompting the goddess Athena to challenge Arachne to a contest. According to the version told by Ovid, Arachne's weaving was not only stunningly beautiful, but depicted all the ways that the gods had abused mortals. Athena was enraged and turned Arachne into a spider and condemned her to weave for evermore, hence the link between ARACHN- and spider.

20. LIMB—border, edge

limbic (LIMB-ic) – pertaining to the edge

circumlimbal (*circum*-LIMB-al) – pertaining to around the edge

The limbic lobe in the brain forms a border around the connection between the two parts of the cerebrum.

21. GYR—circle, coil

gyroidal (GYR-oid-al) – pertaining to shaped like a coil, i.e., spiral

Note that the term gyroidal is unusual in that it has two suffixes.

22. SULC—groove, furrow

sulcate (SULC-ate) – having grooves

sulcal (SULC-al) – pertaining to a groove

The surface of the cerebrum is highly convoluted, with elevated folds and narrow grooves. Each fold is called a gyrus (plural gyri), and each groove is called a sulcus (plural sulci).

23. CINGUL—girdle, belt, structure that surrounds

cingulate (CINGUL-ate) – pertaining to a structure that surrounds

The limbic lobe is sometimes called the cingulate gyrus because it has the form of a curved, encircling layer.

24. AMYGDAL—almond

amygdaloid (AMYGDAL-oid) – resembling an almond

The amygdaloid body is an almond-shaped structure in each temporal lobe. The tonsils are sometimes also called amygdalae because of their almond shape.

25. PITUIT—mucus, phlegm, discharge

pituitary (PITUIT-ary) – pertaining to a discharge

pituitous (PITUIT-ous) – full of mucus

The pituitary gland, located at the base of the brain, got its name because it produces and discharges secretions; these secretions are now known to be hormones.

26. MENT—(i) mind, reason: (ii) chin

mental (MENT-al) – pertaining to the mind, pertaining to the chin

amentia (*a*-MENT-ia) – condition of being without reason or mental capacity

dementia (*de*-MENT-ia) – condition of being out of one's mind, i.e., loss of mental capacity

Though they both have the base MENT-, there is no link between the words for mind and chin. You have to decide from context which of the two is most suitable.

27. PSYCH—mind

psychosis (PSYCH-osis) – abnormal condition of the mind

psychotic (PSYCH-O-tic) – pertaining to the mind

28. THYM—emotion, mind

dysthymia (*dys*-THYM-ia) – condition of difficult emotion, i.e., depression

euthymia (*eu*-THYM-ia) – condition of good emotion

hypothymia (*hypo*-THYM-ia) – condition of less than normal emotion, i.e., depression

hyperthymia (*hyper*-THYM-ia) – condition of more than normal emotion, i.e., mania

Both dysthymia and hypothymia are mood disorders characterized by depression, while hyperthymia is a heightened emotional response that is less intense than a manic disorder. Euthymia represents moderation of mood, neither manic nor depressed. The thymus gland was known to the ancient Greeks, but why they gave it this name is not clear. It may be because of its physical location in the chest, which was thought to be one of the seats of emotion.

29. PHREN—(i) mind: (ii) diaphragm

phrenic (PHREN-ic) – pertaining to the mind, pertaining to the diaphragm

phrenetic (PHREN-etic) – pertaining to the mind, pertaining to the diaphragm

hypophrenia (*hypo*-PHREN-ia) – condition of less than normal mental ability

The phren is a difficult entity to pin down. The ancient Greeks first thought of it as occupying a space around the heart; then it seems to have moved to the midriff area and the diaphragm. However, since both the heart and diaphragm were also associated with the emotions, the concept of the phren was extended to include the mind also. The English words frenetic, frantic, and frenzy are all derived from phren, but with the everyday sense of violent emotions or madness. Ancient Greeks and Romans did believe that an inflammation of the phren produced a serious illness with some symptoms similar to madness.

30. SCHIS—split, division
SCHIST—split, division
SCHIZ—split, division

schizophrenia (SCHIZ-O-PHREN-ia) – condition of a mind that is split

schizencephaly (SCHIZ-ENCEPHAL-y) – state of the brain matter with (abnormal) division

31. SAN—healthy, sound
SANIT—healthy, sound

sanity (SAN-ity) – condition of (being) healthy, usually in regard to mental health

sanitorium (SANIT-orium) – a place for (becoming) healthy

32. MAN—(i) frenzy: (ii) hand: (iii) thin, loose

mania (MAN-ia) – condition of frenzy

hypomania (*hypo*-MAN-ia) – a condition of below frenzy, i.e., a milder form of mania

antimanic (*anti*-MAN-ic) – pertaining to against frenzy, i.e., to counteract mania

This base has three unrelated meanings; we will look at the meanings "hand," and "thin, loose" in later chapters.

33. PRESS—to press, pressing

depression (*de*-PRESS-ion) – condition of downward pressing, i.e., feeling of hopelessness

antidepressive (*anti-de*-PRESS-ive) – pertaining to against downward pressing, i.e., counteracting feeling of hopelessness

Notice here how important context is. If we are discussing someone's mental state, then depression no doubt means a feeling of one's mood being pressed down, i.e., a feeling of hopelessness. However, if we are discussing a type of bone injury, a depression fracture of the skull is one in which the bone fragment presses downward and inward. Notice that antidepressive is unusual in that it has two prefixes.

34. PHOR—to bear, to carry, bearing

euphoria (*eu*-PHOR-ia) – condition of good bearing, i.e., exaggerated happiness

dysphoria (*dys*-PHOR-ia) – condition of difficult bearing, i.e., depression

35. PHOB—fear

phobia (PHOB-ia) – condition of fear

arachnophobic (ARACHN-O-PHOB-ic) – pertaining to a fear of spiders

36. PHIL- loving, affinity to, craving for

dermatophilic (DERMAT-O-PHIL-ic) – pertaining to loving the skin, i.e., pertaining to a product that is supposedly good for the skin

arachnophilia (ARACHN-O-PHIL-ia) – condition of loving spiders

hyperphilia (*hyper*-PHIL-ia) – condition of more than normal craving, i.e., a compulsive desire for sex

37. ANXI—worry

anxious (ANXI-ous) – full of worry

hyperanxiety (*hyper*-ANXI-ety) – condition of more than normal worry

38. MNE—to remember

amnesia (*a*-MNE-sia) – condition of without memory

Many words with the "mn" combination, such as amnesty and mnemonic, have something to do with memory. In Greek mythology, Mnemosyne was the goddess of memory and remembrance, and her name is reflected in words associated with her.

SOME MORE THINGS TO LEARN

Some BASE-suffix pairs occur together so regularly that they are often treated as one suffix. To distinguish them from regular suffixes, we call them compound suffixes. Four examples that you have met in this chapter are MAN-ia, MNES-ia, PHIL-ia, and PHOB-ia, which form the compound suffixes -mania, -mnesia, -philia, and -phobia, respectively. It is helpful to memorize all the compound suffixes, but not absolutely necessary, as you can always build them up from their individual base and suffix parts.

1. -mania	condition of madness, compulsion, obsession
2. -mnesia	condition of memory, memory
3. -philia	condition of attraction, attraction, abnormal craving for
4. -phobia	condition of fear, abnormal fear of

Here are some new bases to learn that can be used with these compound suffixes.

39. ANDR—man, male

andromania (ANDR-O-mania) – obsession about men
androphilia (ANDR-O-philia) – attraction to men
androphobia (ANDR-O-phobia) – abnormal fear of men

40. GYN—woman, female
GYNAEC—woman, female
GYNEC—woman, female

gynophobia (GYN-O-phobia) – abnormal fear of women
gynephilia (GYN-E-philia) – attraction to women
gynecomania (GYNEC-O-mania) – obsession about women

Note the combining vowel in gynephilia is "e."

41. NECR—death, dead

necromania (NECR-O-mania) – obsession about death or dead bodies
necrophilia (NECR-O-philia) – abnormal craving for dead bodies
necrophobia (NECR-O-phobia) – abnormal fear of death or dead bodies

42. XEN—foreign

xenomania (XEN-O-mania) – obsession about foreign things or people
xenophilia (XEN-O-philia – attraction to foreign things or people
xenophobia (XEN-O-phobia) – abnormal fear (or distrust) of foreign things or people

43. PSEUD—false

pseudomnesia (PSEUD-O-mnesia) – memory that is false

44. CRYPT—hidden

cryptomnesia (CRYPT-O-mnesia) – memory that is hidden, i.e., subconscious memory

We saw in Chapter 2 that the suffix -verse is actually made up of the base VERS- and the suffix -e. We can add -verse to the list of compound suffixes, but remember it is unusual because the suffix -e really has no meaning in itself.

5. -verse	to turn, to travel, turned

We have now seen more compound terms that include two bases. Remember, apply the suffix to the ultimate base and make sense of that part of the term first. Then you may be able to apply the suffix to the other base as well, using the word "and" to join the two bases, like we did with temporoparietal, occipitotemporal, and sphenofrontal in this chapter, and dorsoventral in a previous chapter. Sometimes, however, you cannot do this, as we saw with levoversion, caudocephalad, and cephalocaudad earlier. In this chapter, we also came across the terms sphenocephalic, gyrencephalic, schizophrenia, schizencephaly, and arachnophobia and we cannot join the bases with "and" in any of these cases and still make real sense. This is where common sense has to come in again. I suggest always starting your definition off with the ultimate base and its suffix, then think about what extra information the penultimate base could be adding to your definition. Remember, all bases are derived from nouns, adjectives, or verbs, just with their end bits missing. The penultimate base often describes the ultimate base in some way, or it might indicate the circumstance associated with it—how, when, or where. Therefore, our definition order becomes suffix-ULTIMATE BASE-PENULTIMATE BASE. Sometimes, you might end up with a fairly clumsy definition; my definition "pertaining to a brain that has coils," for example, is certainly not elegant, but you can always adjust this afterward if you choose to.

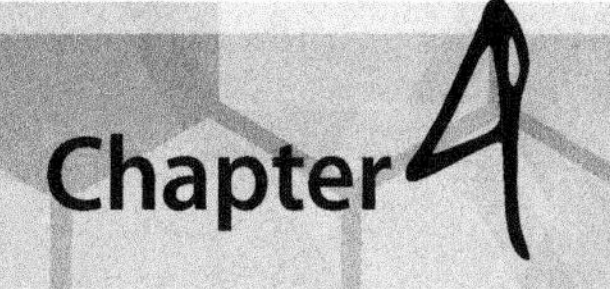

SKIN, HAIR, AND NAILS

PREFIXES

1. *amphi-, ampho-*	both, on both sides
2. *an-*	without, not, non-
3. *dia-*	through, apart, in a line
4. *extra-, extro-*	outside of, beyond
5. *in-*	in, into, over
6. *meta-*	after, change, transition
7. *non-*	not
8. *ob-*	toward, in front of, against
9. *par-*	beside, beyond, abnormal
10. *per-*	through
11. *poly-*	many, much
12. *re-*	again and again, backward
13. *semi-*	half, partly
14. *syn-*	together, with, concurrent

amphi-/ampho- and *extra-/extro-* are just alternative forms of the same prefix.

SUFFIXES

1. -aceous	pertaining to, belonging to, having
2. -atic	pertaining to
3. -ation	process
4. -atory	pertaining to
5. -cle	small
6. -cyte	cell
7. -escent	beginning to be, becoming
8. -esis	condition, abnormal condition, process
9. -gen	that which produces
10. -in	substance
11. -ment	action of, product of
12. -oma	tumor, mass
13. -ose	full of, having the quality of
14. -ula	small
15. -um	structure, substance

BASES

First, some bases relating to the skin and to the tissue immediately below it (the subcutaneous tissues). Remember, we saw in Chapter 2 the bases DERM- and DERMAT- also mean skin. Make sure that you have learned them.

1. CUT—skin
CUTANE—skin

cuticle (CUT-I-cle) – small skin, i.e., an edge of skin covering the nail bed, or a thin layer of skin

cutaneous (CUTANE-ous) – pertaining to the skin

subcutaneous (*sub*-CUTANE-ous) – pertaining to below the skin

extracutaneous (*extra*-CUTANE-ous) – pertaining to outside of the skin, i.e., not affecting the skin

Note the combining vowel in cuticle is "i." We have two bases meaning "skin," DERM-/DERMAT- and CUT-/CUTANE-; as we have seen previously, this is because one term has been derived from Greek, and the other from Latin.

2. **TECT—to cover**
   TEG—to cover

tectorium (TECT-orium) – a place for covering, i.e., a covering structure or layer

integument (*in*-TEG-U-ment) – product of over covering, i.e., something that covers or encloses, especially a skin or membrane

This base provides another common name for the skin, the integument or integumentary layer. Note the combining vowel in integument is "u."

3. **SARC—flesh, soft tissue**

sarcoma (SARC-oma) – tumor of the soft tissues

sarcoid (SARC-oid) – resembling flesh

In medicine, SARC- generally relates to the muscular and connective tissues. A sarcoma is a malignant (cancerous) tumor. Sarcoid was, at one time, also a term for a tumor similar to a sarcoma; hence this term, which is still in use:

sarcoidosis (SARC-oid-osis) – abnormal condition of tumors of the soft tissues (it also affects many different organs of the body, and even the bones of the feet and hands)

Note that the term sarcoidosis is unusual in that it has two suffixes.

4. **THEL—(i) nipple: (ii) cellular layer, tissue**

epithelium (*epi*-THEL-I-um) – structure on the surface tissue, i.e., a tissue that covers all surfaces, including the skin (where it called the epidermis)

Although this base means "nipple," you will rarely come across it in this context. Back in the 17th century, when no other suitable Greek or Latin term could be found, its meaning was extended to mean a cellular layer or tissue. Not everyone agreed with the choice, as you can read about in later medical discussions, but the term stuck. Notice that the combing vowel in epithelium is "i."

5. **CYT—cell**

    cytoid (CYT-oid) – resembling a cell

Remember that we saw that the base VERS- plus the suffix -e formed a new suffix -verse. Well, a similar thing happens with the base CYT-. When the suffix -e is added to it, it forms the suffix -cyte; we can think of it as a compound suffix. Remember, the suffix -e does not have a meaning of its own.

6. **HIST—tissue**
   HISTI—tissue

    histoid (HIST-oid) – resembling tissue

    histiocyte (HISTI-O-cyte) – cell within tissue, i.e., an immune cell that destroys foreign substance that remains within the tissue

7. **KERAT—(i) horn, horny tissue: (ii) cornea (of the eye)**

    keratin (KERAT-in) – substance (composed of) horny tissue, i.e., a hard, fibrous protein

    keratosis (KERAT-osis) – abnormal condition of the horny tissue

    keratoid (KERAT-oid) – resembling horny tissue, resembling corneal tissue

Keratin is the main structural component of the outer layer of the skin (epidermis), as well as the hair, nails, and the cornea of the eye.

8. **MELAN—black**

    melanin (MELAN-in) – substance that is black

More specifically, melanin is a dark pigment that occurs in the outer layer of the skin, the hair, and the colored part of the eye.

9. **COLL—glue**

    colloid (COLL-oid) – like glue

    collagen (COLL-A-gen) – that which produces glue

Collagen is a major protein in the white fibers of connective tissue. When it is boiled down, it produces gelatin, a gluelike substance. Note the combining vowel in collagen is "a."

10. **ELAST—flexible, stretchy**

    elastin (ELAST-in) – substance that is stretchy

    elastoma (ELAST-oma) – a mass composed of elastic (tissue)

    nonelastic (*non*-ELAST-ic) – pertaining to not flexible

Elastin is a major protein of connective tissues in flexible structures such as the large blood vessels, tendons, and ligaments. Both collagen and elastin are found in the lower level of the skin (dermis).

11. SUD—sweat
SUDOR—sweat

sudation (SUD-ation) – process of sweating

sudoresis (SUDOR-esis) – abnormal condition of sweating

12. FER—to bear, to carry, to produce

dorsiferous (DORS-I-FER-ous) – pertaining to carrying on the back

sudoriferous (SUDOR-I-FER-ous) – pertaining to producing sweat

Sweating occurs through the sudoriferous glands located in the lower level of the skin. Note the combining vowel in both of these terms is "i."

13. HIDR—sweat

synhidrosis (*syn*-HIDR-osis) – condition of concurrent sweating, i.e., the association of sweating along with some other symptom

anhidrosis (*an*-HIDR-osis) – condition of without sweat, i.e., the inability to sweat normally

We met the prefix *a*-, meaning without, not, previously in the term amnesia. Here, it takes the form *an*- because it precedes the letter "h." There are several prefixes that have alternative forms depending on whether they go before a base starting with a consonant, or one starting with a vowel or the letter "h." This is explained further in the some things to note section. Both of the bases SUD- and HIDR- mean sweat; again, this is because one term has been derived from Greek and the other from Latin. Diaphoresis (*dia*-PHOR-esis) also means sweating; if we break the term apart, it literally means "condition of through carrying." The act of sweating can also be termed perspiration:

14. SPIR—(i) to breathe: (ii) coil

perspiration (*per*-SPIR-ation) – process of through breathing, i.e., excretion through (the skin)

respiratory (*re*-SPIR-atory) – pertaining to again and again breathing, i.e., the continual process of breathing

spiroid (SPIR-oid) – resembling a coil

SPIR- has two unconnected meanings, "to breathe" and "coil." You have to decide from context which of the two is most suitable.

15. LIP—fat

lipocyte (LIP-O-cyte) – cell containing fat

lipoma (LIP-oma) – tumor containing fat (cells)

16. ADIP—fat

adiposis (ADIP-osis) – abnormal condition of fat (deposit), i.e., obesity

adipose (ADIP-ose) – full of fat

17. STEAR—fat
STEAT—fat

stearic (STEAR-ic) – pertaining to fat

steatosis (STEAT-osis) – abnormal condition of fat (deposit)

We have three bases here that all mean fat, two derived from Greek and one from Latin. The subcutaneous tissue lies immediately below the skin; one of its major purposes is to store fat that functions as an energy reserve, and as an insulating and protective layer. The fat is stored in adipose tissue containing adipocytes or lipocytes (both terms are in use).

Now some bases related to the hair and nails:

18. TRICH—hair

schizotrichia (SCHIZ-O-TRICH-ia) – condition of hair that is split (at the ends)

melanotrichous (MELAN-O-TRICH-ous) – pertaining to hair that is black

amphitrichous (*amphi*-TRICH-ous) – pertaining to on both sides hair, i.e., hair, or hairlike structures, at both ends

This last term, amphitrichous, is a bit awkward to define in the order that we have been using, suffix-*prefix*-BASE, but, if you think about it, it still makes sense and you can adjust your final definition to something closer to normal English.

19. PIL—hair

pilose (PIL-ose) – full of hair, i.e., hairy

piliferous (PIL-I-FER-ous) – pertaining to bearing or producing hair

depilation (*de*-PIL-ation) – process of without hair, i.e., process for removal of hair

Note the combining vowel in piliferous is “i.”

20. MEDULL—innermost part, medulla

medullary (MEDULL-ary) – pertaining to the innermost part

21. CORT—outer layer, cortex
CORTIC—outer layer, cortex

cortical (CORTIC-al) – pertaining to the outer layer

22. FOLL—sac, container

follicle (FOLL-I-cle) – small sac, i.e., a small cavity or sac

Derived from the term for a bellow or leather purse, a follicle is a group of cells that contain a small cavity or sac; another structure often grows within the cavity. Every hair on the human body grows within a hair follicle. Note the combining vowel in follicle is "i." The hair itself is composed of three layers: an inner medulla and an outer cortex, covered by the cuticle, and a layer of dead cells containing keratin.

23. SEB—grease, tallow

sebum (SEB-um) – substance (that is like) grease, i.e., sebum

sebaceous (SEB-aceous) – pertaining to grease, i.e., pertaining to sebum

Sebum is secreted by sebaceous glands in the skin onto the hair shaft to lubricate and protect it.

24. UNGU—nail

ungual (UNGU-al) – pertaining to a nail or nails

unguiferate (UNGU-I-FER-ate) – pertaining to bearing nails

polyunguia (*poly*-UNGU-ia) – condition of many nails, i.e., having extra nails on fingers or toes

Note the combining vowel in unguiferate is "i."

25. ONYCH—nail

paronychia (*par*-ONYCH-ia) – condition beside the nail, i.e., an infection of the skin just next to the nail

polyonychia (*poly*-ONYCH-ia) – condition of many nails, i.e., having extra nails on fingers or toes

melanonychia (MELAN-ONYCH-ia) – condition of a nail that is black

The prefix *par*- in paronychia is the alternative form of the prefix *para*-, which you have not met yet, used here because the base that follows begins with a vowel; see some more things to learn below.

26. LUN—moon, moon shaped

lunate (LUN-ate) – pertaining to moon shaped

semilunar (*semi*-LUN-ar) – pertaining to half moon shaped

lunula (LUN-ula) – small moon, i.e., the crescent moon shaped whitish area of the nail

When meaning "moon shaped," LUN- almost always means crescent shaped, like a crescent moon. The base LUN- also gave rise to the English terms lunacy and lunatic, since it was once believed that madness was influenced by the phases of the moon.

SOME MORE THINGS TO LEARN

We saw above that the prefix *an-* is just a modified form of the prefix *a-* that we had met previously. The form *an-* is used when the following base begins with a vowel, or the letter "h." This is done to avoid hiatus, the slight pause that occurs when two vowel sounds are next to each other without a consonant between them. This does not happen only with *a-*; many of the Greek prefixes that end with a vowel have alternative forms to use before bases that begin with vowels or the letter "h." Usually, this involves dropping off the final vowel of the prefix (unlike *a-*, which adds on an "n"). This process is known as elision. We do something similar in the English language when we shorten "I am" to "I'm" or "you are" to "you're," although we actually elide the vowel of the following word. Note, however, that the practice is inconsistent; sometimes elision does occur, sometimes it does not, even with a prefix that normally undergoes elision. In general, Latin prefixes do not elide. From now on, the list of prefixes you have to learn will include any alternative forms. Here are the prefixes that you have already met that are included in this type:

1. *a-, an-*	not, without, non-
2. *anti-, ant-*	against, opposite
3. *apo-, ap-*	away from
4. *dia-, di-*	through, apart, in a line
5. *ecto-, ect-*	outside, outer
6. *endo-, end-*	inside, inner
7. *epi-, ep-*	upon, on the surface
8. *hypo-, hyp-*	below, deficient, less than normal
9. *meta-, met-*	after, change, transition
10. *para-, par-*	beside, beyond, abnormal

Note that the alternative form of *dia-* still ends in a vowel. The prefix *peri-* never elides, so there is no possibility of confusing it with the prefix *per-*.

We have now seen several instances of different bases meaning the same thing, often because we have bases derived from both Greek and Latin languages. Occasionally, both bases can be combined with the same suffix to create terms with the same meaning, as we saw with steatosis and adiposis, but this is not common and you should not rely on this being the case.

The skin, hair, and nails are often described by their color. We saw the base MELAN- meaning "black" above; here are some more bases that indicate color for you to memorize:

27. CHRO—color
CHROM—color
CHROMAT—color

metachroic (*meta*-CHRO-ic) – pertaining to change in color

dyschromia (*dys*-CHROM-ia) – condition of abnormal color, i.e., discoloration, especially of skin or nails

achromatic (*a*-CHROMAT-ic) – pertaining to without color

28. NIGR—black

nigrescent (NIGR-escent) – beginning to be black

29. ALB—white
ALBID—white, whitish

albescent (ALB-escent) – beginning to be white

People suffering from albinism lack pigment in the skin, hair, and eyes (or, the eyes only), caused by abnormal melanin production. You may come across the terms albicans and nigricans, meaning "whitish" and "blackish," respectively.

30. LEUC—white
LEUK—white

leukotrichia (LEUK-O-TRICH-ia) – condition of hair that is white

leukocyte (LEUK-O-cyte) – cell that is white, i.e., a white (blood) cell

The alternative spelling LEUC- (where the "k" of the Greek form is replaced by "c") is occasionally used.

31. CAN—white, gray
CAND—white, glowing white

canescent (CAN-escent) – beginning to be white or gray

A term you might come across in relation to hair is canities, which means whiteness or grayness of the hair due to diminishing pigment.

32. POLI—gray

trichopoliosis (TRICH-O-POLI-osis) – condition of graying of the hair

This base can also be found in terms relating to the gray matter of the central nervous system (the nerve cell structures that are not coated with the white lipoprotein myelin), as opposed to the white matter (the nerve cell structures that are coated with the white lipoprotein myelin).

33. ERYTHR—red

erythrodermic (ERYTHR-O-DERM-ic) – pertaining to skin that is red

erythrocyte (ERYTHR-O-cyte) – cell that is red, i.e., a red blood cell

34. RUB—red
RUBR—red

rubeosis (RUB-E-osis) – condition of red (discoloration of the skin)

rubricyte (RUBR-I-cyte) – cell that is red, i.e., a red blood cell (in an immature stage)

Note the combining vowels "e" and "i."

35. ROSE—rosy-red, pink

roseate (ROSE-ate) – having rosy-red (coloration)

36. RHOD—rosy-red

rhodescent (RHOD-escent) – beginning to be rosy-red

The metal rhodium is not itself rosy-red, but one of the salts from which the first extractions of the metal were made is; this prompted its discoverer to name the new element after the Greek for rose. The light-sensitive pigment in the eye, commonly known as visual purple, is called rhodopsin, and appears reddish-purple.

37. PURPUR—purple

purpuric (PURPUR-ic) – pertaining to a purple (condition), i.e., pertaining to purpura, a condition that at one stage is characterize by a purple discoloration of the skin

purpuriferous (PURPUR-I-FER-ous) – pertaining to producing (visual) purple

Note the combining vowel "i."

38. PORPHYR—purple

porphyrin (PORPHYR-in) – substance that is purple

porphyria (PORPHYR-ia) – condition of purple, i.e., the condition porphyria

Porphyrins are naturally occurring organic compounds, many of which are characterized by their purple color. In the condition porphyria, excessive excretion of porphyrins can result in urine and feces that turn purple when exposed to the air, or in purple lesions on the skin.

39. FUSC—brown, dark

fuscin (FUSC-in) – substance that is brown, i.e., a brown pigment in the retina of the eye

obfuscate (*ob*-FUSC-ate) – to cause to (bring) toward darkness, i.e., to cause things to be unclear

40. CIRRH—yellow, tawny

cirrhosis (CIRRH-osis) – condition of yellow (discoloration)

The term cirrhosis originated with the yellow discoloration of a diseased liver. We generally call the yellow discoloration of the skin that occurs through liver degeneration jaundice, a term derived from the French language, although we will meet a base meaning jaundice in a later chapter.

41. FLAV—golden yellow, reddish-yellow

flavin (FLAV-in) – substance that is reddish-yellow, i.e., a variety of yellow pigment

You might just come across the term flavedo; it is quite outdated now, but it means a yellowing of the skin.

42. LUTE—yellow

lutein (LUTE-in) – substance that is yellow, i.e., a chemical substance isolated from egg yolk

You will most likely come across this base in relation to the corpus luteum, literally the "yellow body," a structure formed in the ovary after ovulation:

luteal (LUTE-al) – pertaining to the corpus luteum

43. XANTH—yellow

xanthosis (XANTH-osis) – condition of yellowing (of the skin)

44. CHLOR—green

chlorosis (CHLOR-osis) – condition of green (discoloration of the skin)

The gas chlorine got its name because of its yellow-green color. You will find the base CHLOR- meaning "chlorine" in many chemical terms.

45. GLAUC—bluish-gray, silvery-gray

glaucescent (GLAUC-escent) – beginning to be bluish-gray

Most of the terms you will come across using this base relate to the condition glaucoma, an eye disease referred to by the ancient Greeks. Why they named it this is unclear; it may refer to a bluish-gray haze seen in the pupil of an affected eye, although this is more likely indicative of cataracts than the condition glaucoma as we understand it today.

46. CYAN—blue

cyanosis (CYAN-osis) – condition of blue (discoloration of the skin)

Some other color-related bases that you might come across, though not very often, are TEPHR- and CINER-/CINE-, both of which actually mean "ashes," but are used in terminology to indicate the color of ashes, i.e., gray. Likewise PHAEO-/PHEO-, literally the "color of the sky at twilight," is used for gray or dusky, while EOSIN-, the "color of the sky at dawn," indicates a rosy-red hue.

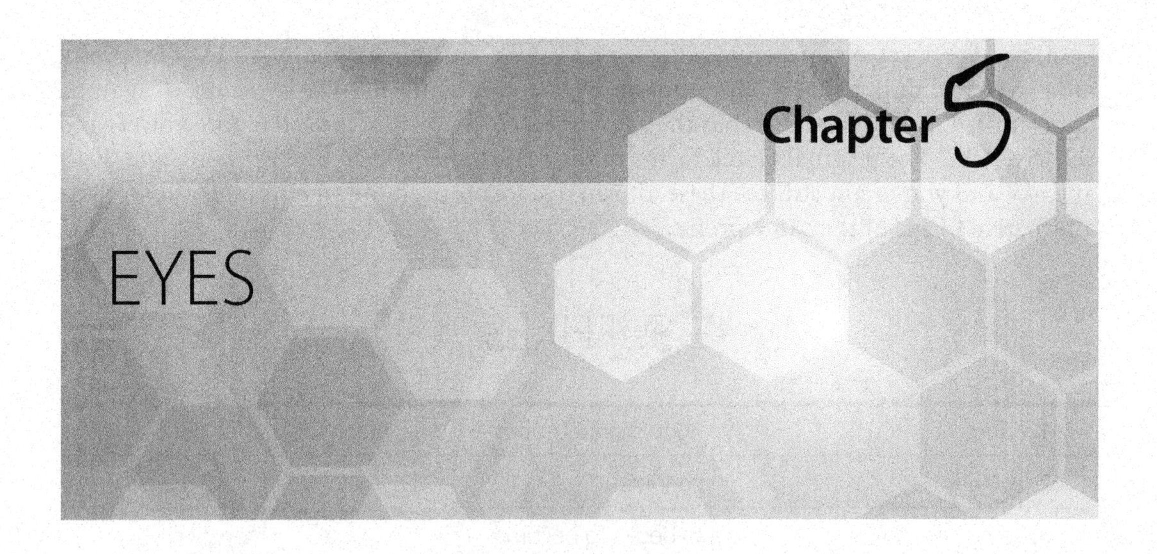

Chapter 5

EYES

PREFIXES

1. *ante-*	before, in front of
2. *cata-, cat-*	down, complete
3. *con-*	together, with
4. *ec-, ex-*	out, outside
5. *eiso-, eso-*	inward,
6. *ento-, ent-*	inside, within
7. *hemi-*	half
8. *infra-*	below
9. *multi-*	many, much
10. *post-*	behind, after
11. *pros-*	toward
12. *supra-*	above

Note the forms *cata-/cat-* and *ento-/ent-*; these two prefixes have alternative forms depending on whether the base that follows begins with a consonant, or with a vowel or the letter "h." Remember, elision does not occur with all prefixes that end in a vowel;

here, the final vowels of *hemi-*, *infra-*, and *supra-* do not normally elide. The prefix *ante-* never elides, so there is no possibility of confusing it with *anti-/ant-* ("against, opposite"). The prefix *ec-* also has the alternative form *ex-* that is used before vowels and the letter "h." The original Greek forms of the prefixes *cata-/cat-* and *ec-* were *kata-/kat-* and *ek-*, and you might still see these alternative forms used today. *eiso-* and *eso-* are just alternative forms of the same prefix.

SUFFIXES

1. -duct	duct, channel, tube
2. -ema	condition
3. -esce	to begin, to become
4. -form	having the form of, like
5. -gram	record
6. -graph	instrument used to record
7. -iasis	state of, process of, abnormal condition
8. -iatic	pertaining to a state, pertaining to a process
9. -ible, -ibil-	able to be
10. -ical	pertaining to
11. -itis	inflammation
12. -ize	to make, to affect
13. -meter	instrument used to measure
14. -scope	instrument used to examine
15. -ual	pertaining to

Note that when the suffix -ible is combined with another suffix after it, its form changes to -ibil-. So, for example, visible (VIS-ible), but visibility (VIS-ibil-ity).

BASES

We have seen previously that different bases can have the same meaning. This is also true for some of the bases here related to the eye and sight, and for many of the bases we will encounter in the remaining chapters. Be sure to memorize all forms.

1. **PHOT—light**

   photodermatitis (PHOT-O-DERMAT-itis) – inflammation of the skin (caused by exposure to) light

   photoerythema (PHOT-O-ERYTH-ema) – condition of reddening (of the skin due to) light

   photometer (PHOT-O-meter) – instrument to measure light

2. **SCOT—darkness**

   scotosis (SCOT-osis) – abnormal condition of darkness (in the visual field), i.e., a blind spot

   scotophobia (SCOT-O-phobia) – abnormal fear of the darkness

3. **BLEP—to see, sight**
   BLEPS—to see, sight

   ablepsia (*a*-BLEPS-ia) – condition of without sight, i.e., blindness

   parablepsy (*para*-BLEPS-y) – state of beyond (normal) sight, i.e., hallucination, visual illusion

4. **VID—to see, sight**
   VIS—to see, sight

   visual (VIS-ual) – pertaining to seeing or sight

   visible (VIS-ible) – able to be seen

   visibility (VIS-ibil-ity) – state of being able to be seen

   xenovision (XEN-O-VIS-ion) – act of seeing strange or foreign (things in the imagination)

Note the change in the form of the suffix -ible to -ibil- in the term visibility, due to the combination of the two suffixes.

5. **OP—eye, sight**
   OPS—eye, sight
   OPT—eye, sight

   scotopia (SCOT-OP-ia) – process of sight in the dark, i.e., the adaptation of the eye to seeing in the dark hemianopsia (*hemi-an*-OPS-ia) – condition of half non-sight, i.e., loss of vision in half the visual field

entoptic (*ent*-OPT-ic) – pertaining to within the eye

optomeningeal (OPT-O-MENING-eal) – pertaining to the membrane of the eye, i.e., pertaining to the retina

Note that the term hemianopsia is unusual in that it has two prefixes (actually, we will find it is unusual in another way later on). Remember, we use the prefix *an-* instead of *a-* (meaning "not, without, non-") when the following base begins with a vowel or the letter "h." When the base OP- is combined with the prefix *pros-*, we get the new base PROSOP-:

6. **PROSOP—face**

   prosopic (PROSOP-ic) – pertaining to the face

7. **OCUL—eye, sight**

   infraocular (*infra*-OCUL-ar) – pertaining to below the eye

   oculofacial (OCUL-O-FACI-al) – pertaining to the face and eyes

   postocular (*post*-OCUL-ar) – pertaining to behind the eye

8. **OPHTHALM—eye, sight**

   exophthalmic (*ex*-OPHTHALM-ic) – pertaining to an outward eye, i.e., pertaining to an abnormal protrusion of the eyeball from the socket

   xenophthalmia (XEN-OPHTHALM-ia) condition of the eye (caused by a) foreign (body)

   anophthalmia (*an*-OPHTHALM-ia) – condition of without eyes

   ophthalmoscope (OPHTHALM-O-scope) – instrument to examine the eyes

   ophthalmograph (OPHTHALM-O-graph) – instrument used to record (movement) of the eyes

Note that the prefix *ex-* is the alternative form of *ec-* that is used before vowels and the letter "h."

9. **ORBIT—wheel track, circle, ring**

   orbital (ORBIT-al) – pertaining to a circular (path)

The base ORBIT- has been given a specific meaning that relates to the orbit of the eye (the eye socket), the bony cavity that contains the eyeball and associated parts:

ORBIT—orbit (of the eye)

anteorbital (*ante*-ORBIT-al) – pertaining to in front of the orbit of the eye

orbitotemporal (ORBIT-O-TEMPOR-al) – pertaining to the temporal and orbital bones and regions

supraorbital (*supra*-ORBIT-al) – pertaining to above the orbit of the eye

10. BLEPHAR—eyelid

ablephary (*a*-BLEPHAR-y) – state of without eyelids

symblepharosis (*sym*-BLEPHAR-osis) – abnormal condition of together eyelids, i.e., the upper and lower eyelids stuck together, or to the eyeball

blepharogram (BLEPHAR-O-gram) – record of eyelid (movement), i.e., the trace on a graph that records the eyelid movement

11. PALPEBR—eyelid

postpalpebral (*post*-PALPEBR-al) – pertaining to behind the eyelid

palpebrate (PALPEBR-ate) – having eyelids

palpebration (PALPEBR-ation) – process with the eyelid, i.e., winking

12. GEN—to produce, to beget
GENIT—to produce, to beget

genesis (GEN-esis) – process of production

adipogenic (ADIP-O-GEN-ic) – pertaining to production of fat

metagenesis (*meta*-GEN-esis) – process of transitional production, i.e., alternation of generations

genital (GENIT-al) – pertaining to reproduction

13. CILI—eyelid, eyelash, hairlike structures

ciliary (CILI-ary) – pertaining to the eyelid or eyelashes

ciliogenesis (CILI-O-GEN-esis) – process of production of eyelashes or hairlike structures

multiciliate (*multi*-CILI-ate) – having many hairlike structures

The ciliary body of the eye is actually within the eyeball itself; it contains muscles that can change the shape of the eye lens.

14. JUNCT—to join

conjunctive (*con*-JUNCT-ive) – pertaining to together joined, i.e., joining, connecting

We get the term conjunctiva from this base, the name for the delicate membrane that lines the eyelid and covers part of the surface of the eyeball, in effect connecting the eyelid and eyeball. We can think of CONJUNCTIV- as a base:

15. CONJUNCTIV—conjunctiva (membrane of the eye)

conjunctival (CONJUCTIV-al) – pertaining to the conjunctiva

conjunctivitis (CONJUNCTIV-itis) – inflammation of the conjunctiva

conjunctivoma (CONJUNCTIV-oma) – tumor of the conjunctiva

16. SCLER—hard, firm, thick

sclerodermal (SCLER-O-DERM-al) – pertaining to skin that is hard or thick

scleronychia (SCLER-ONYCH-ia) – condition of hardening or thickening of the nails

We get the term sclera from this base, the name for the firm outer coating of the eyeball:

SCLER—sclera (the white of the eye)

scleritis (SCLER-itis) – inflammation of the sclera

17. CORN—horn
CORNE—horn

corneous (CORNE-ous) – pertaining to horn

cornual (CORN-ual) – pertaining to horn

We saw in the previous chapter that the base KERAT-, "horn," was related to the cornea of the eye, since parts of the cornea contain the hard, fibrous protein keratin; likewise, the base CORN-/CORNE-, also meaning "horn," relates to the cornea:

CORNE—cornea (of the eye)

corneal (CORNE-al) – pertaining to the cornea

corneoscleral (CORNE-O-SCLER-al) – pertaining to the sclera and cornea

18. RET—net, network

retiform (RET-I-form) – like a net

Note the combining vowel in retiform is "i." We get the term retina from this base, the name for the photo-sensitive layer of the eye characterized by a network of blood vessels. We can think of RETIN- as a base:

19. RETIN—retina (of the eye)

retinitis (RETIN-itis) – inflammation of the retina

retinosis (RETIN-osis) – abnormal condition of the retina

retinoschisal (RETIN-O-SCHIS-al) – pertaining to a split or rupture within the retina

20. CHOR—membrane
CHORI—membrane

choroid (CHOR-oid) – like a membrane

chorioid (CHORI-oid) – like a membrane

Two specific membranes related to this base are the chorion, one of the fetal membranes, and the choroid, a membrane that is part of the internal structure of the eye:

CHORI—chorion, choroid
CHORION—chorion
CHOROID—choroid

chorionic (CHORION-ic) – pertaining to the chorion

choroidal (CHOROID-al) – pertaining to the choroid

choroiditis (CHOROID-itis) – inflammation of the choroid

21. TROCH—wheel, round shaped, pulley shaped
TROCHLE—pulley shaped

trochoid (TROCH-oid) – like a wheel, i.e., revolving or rotating

trochocephalia (TROCH-O-CEPHAL-ia) – condition of the head that is (abnormally) round shaped, i.e., an abnormally round head due to premature fusion of the cranial bones

We get the term trochlea from this base, the name for any structure in which a loop acts like a pulley for a tendon to run through, or a grooved structure that acts like a pulley wheel. In the eye, the trochlea is a fibrous loop in the eye orbit through which the tendons of the eye muscles pass:

TROCHLE—trochlea

trochlear (TROCHLE-ar) – pertaining to a trochlea

trochleiform (TROCHLE-I-form) – like a trochlea

Note the combining vowel in trochleiform is "i."

22. CYST—bladder, cyst, sac

cystitis (CYST-itis) – inflammation of the (urinary) bladder

cystic (CYST-ic) – pertaining to a bladder, cyst or sac

23. PHAC—(i) lentil bean: (ii) eye lens
PHAK—(i) lentil bean: (ii) eye lens

phacoid (PHAC-oid) – resembling a lentil bean, resembling an eye lens

phakoma (PHAK-oma) – tumor associated with the eye lens

phacocystic (PHAC-O-CYST-ic) – pertaining to the sac (containing) the eye lens

The phacocyst (the sac containing the eye lens) is more commonly called the lens capsule.

24. LENT—(i) lentil bean: (ii) eye lens
LENTICUL—(i) lentil bean: (ii) eye lens

lentiform (LENT-I-form) – having the form of a lentil bean, having the form of an eye lens

lenticular (LENTICUL-ar) – pertaining to a lentil, pertaining to a lens

In both Greek and Latin, the eye lens got its name because it resembles a lentil bean in shape and size. Note the combining vowel in lentiform is "i." The base LENTICUL- is actually a diminutive form of LENT-, meaning "small lentil, small lens."

25. IRID—rainbow
IRIS—rainbow

iridesce (IRID-esce) – to become like a rainbow, i.e., having rainbowlike colors

We get the term for the iris of the eye from this base. In Greek mythology, Iris was the goddess of the rainbow and messenger of the gods. Supposedly, the iris of the eye got its name because, like the rainbow, it can be many different colors.

IRID—iris (colored portion of the eye)
IRIS—iris (colored portion of the eye)

iridesis (IRID-esis) – abnormal condition of the iris

iridoschisal (IRID-O-SCHIS-al) – pertaining to a split or rupture within the iris

irisopsia (IRIS-OPS-ia) – condition of seeing rainbow colors (around objects)

26. UV—grape

uviform (UV-I-form) – like a grape

uvula (UV-ula) – small grape, i.e., uvula, a small grapelike structure

Note the combining vowel in uviform is "i." The term uvula generally refers to the pendulous mass at the back of the mouth that shows some resemblance to a small grape on a stem. We can think of UVUL- as a base:

27. UVUL—uvula

uvulitis (UVUL-itis) – inflammation of the uvula

In the eye, the iris, ciliary body, and the choroid are collectively called the uvea. The term derives from this base for grape, presumably due to some similarities in size and appearance between the two. We can think of UVE- as a base:

28. UVE—uvea

uveal (UVE-al) – pertaining to the uvea

uveitis (UVE-itis) – inflammation of the uvea

uveomeningitis (UVE-O-MENING-itis) – inflammation of the meninges and the uvea

29. STEN—narrow, contracted

dermostenosis (DERM-O-STEN-osis) – condition of contraction of the skin

sclerostenosis (SCLER-O-STEN-osis) – condition of contraction caused by hardening or thickening (of tissue)

stenophobia (STEN-O-phobia) – abnormal fear of narrow (spaces)

30. TON—tone, tension, stretching

tonia (TON-ia) – condition of tone, i.e., normal condition of tone or tension in a muscle

atony (*a*-TON-y) – quality of without tone, i.e., quality of a muscle that has lost its strength or firmness

hypertonic (*hyper*-TON-ic) – pertaining to more than normal tone or tension, i.e., pertaining to a muscle in a state of extreme tension, causing inability to stretch

catatonia (*cata*-TON-ia) – condition of complete tension, i.e., a complete rigidity of the muscles resulting in lack of mobility, a symptom of a particular behavioral abnormality or mental impairment

31. COR—pupil (of the eye)
CORE—pupil (of the eye)

dyscoria (*dys*-COR-ia) – condition of abnormal pupil or pupils

stenocoriasis (STEN-O-COR-iasis) – state of the pupil marked by narrowing, i.e., constriction of the pupil

32. PUPILL—pupil

interpupillary (*inter*-PUPILL-ary) – pertaining to between the pupils, i.e., generally pertaining to the distance between the pupils

pupillatonia (PUPILL-*a*-TON-ia) – condition of without tone in the pupil, i.e., the pupil lacks the ability to contract

Both Greek and Latin terms for the pupil derive from words for a little doll or puppet, since, supposedly, if you look into someone's pupil, you see a puppetlike reflection of yourself. The term pupillatonia is unusual in that there is a base preceding the prefix.

33. LACRIM—tears

lacrimatory (LACRIM-atory) – pertaining to tears

lacrimal (LACRIM-al) – pertaining to tears

lacrimation (LACRIM-ation) – process of (producing) tears

34. DACRY—tears

dacryogenic (DACRY-O-GEN-ic) – pertaining to producing tears

dacryocystic (DACRY-O-CYST-ic) – pertaining to the sac related to tears, i.e., pertaining to the lacrimal sac

dacryocystitis (DACRY-O-CYST-itis) – inflammation of the sac related to tears, i.e., inflammation of the lacrimal sac

35. VITR—glass
VITRE—glass

vitric (VITR-ic) – pertaining to glass

vitreous (VITRE-ous) – like glass

One specific use of this base is in the term vitreous humor, the gelatinous, glasslike fluid between the lens and retina in the eye:

VITR—vitreous humor
VITRE—vitreous humor

vitritis (VITR-itis) – inflammation of the vitreous humor

vitreoretinal (VITRE-O-RETIN-al) – pertaining to the retina and the vitreous humor

36. HYAL—glass

hyalophobia (HYAL-O-phobia) – abnormal fear of glass (objects)

hyaloid (HYAL-oid) – resembling glass, i.e., glassy, translucent appearance

Like VITR- and VITRE-, this base is also used about the gelatinous, glasslike fluid between the lens and retina in the eye:

HYAL—vitreous humor

hyalitis (HYAL-itis) – inflammation of the vitreous humor

hyalosis (HYAL-osis) – abnormal condition of the vitreous humor

37. AQU—water, watery fluid
AQUE—water, watery fluid

aquaphobia (AQU-A-phobia) – abnormal fear of water

aqueduct (AQUE-duct) – a duct or channel that carries water

aqueous (AQUE-ous) – like water, i.e., watery

Note the combining vowel in aquaphobia is "a." The aqueous humor is the watery fluid between the lens and cornea in the eye.

38. MEI—lesser, smaller
MI—lesser, smaller

meiosis (MEI-osis) – process of making lesser, i.e., process of cell division in which the number of chromosomes is lessened

miosis (MI-osis) – process of making smaller, i.e., process of constriction (of the pupil)

miotic (MI-O-tic) – pertaining to the process of miosis

The opposite of miosis of the pupil is mydriasis, a widening of the pupil.

39. MYOP—shortsighted, nearsighted

myopia (MYOP-ia) – condition of nearsightedness

myopic (MYOP-ic) – pertaining to nearsightedness

This base originates from the Greek meaning "contracted eye," since those who are shortsighted often partly close their eyes, or squint, in order to try and focus on distant objects. The opposite condition is hyperopia (*hyper*-OP-ia), literally "condition of more than normal sight," or farsightedness, in which sufferers have difficulty focusing on near objects.

40. TROP—to turn, turning

phototropic (PHOT-O-TROP-ic) – pertaining to turning (in response) to the light

esotropia (*eso*-TROP-ia) – condition of inward turning, i.e., a condition of the eyes in which one or both eyes turn inward

SOME MORE THINGS TO LEARN

In Chapter 3, we noted that some base-suffix pairs occur together so regularly that they are often treated as one compound suffix. There we saw -phobia, -philia, -mania, and -mnesia; here we will look at some more. First, three that use some of the bases we have just learned:

1. -blepsia	condition of sight
2. -opia	condition of sight
3. -opsia	condition of sight

Now, three others compound suffixes using new bases (these new bases need to be memorized):

41. GRAPH—to write, to record

dysgraphia (*dys*-GRAPH-ia) – condition of bad or difficult writing, i.e., inability to write

42. METR—(i) measurement: (ii) womb, uterus

metrical (METR-ical) – pertaining to measurement

metricize (METR-ic-ize) – to make pertaining to measurement

Note that the term metricize is unusual in that it has two suffixes. We will come back to METR- meaning "womb, uterus" in a later chapter.

43. SCOP—to view, to examine

optoscopic (OPTO-SCOP-ic) – pertaining to examination of the eye

All three of these bases are regularly combined with the suffix -y to form -graphy, -metry, and -scopy:

4. -graphy	process of recording
5. -metry	process of measuring
6. -scopy	process of examining with an instrument

We have already seen how the final vowel of some prefixes gets dropped when the prefix is added to a base beginning with a vowel or the letter "h." We called this process elision. Something similar happens with some prefixes that end in a consonant; however, in this case, the change occurs when the following base also begins with a consonant. The six prefixes that we have met so far that this applies to are *con-*, *en-*, *in-*, *syn-*, *ob-*, and *sub-*. When they go before bases that begin with certain consonants, the final consonant of the prefix changes to something closer to the beginning consonant of the base. This happens because, in speaking, the tongue anticipates what sound is coming next. This process is called assimilation, with the consonants similar or identical to each other.

Therefore, for *con-*,

when the base begins with l, *con-* becomes *col-*
when the base begins with b, *con-* becomes *com-*
when the base begins with m, *con-* becomes *com-*
when the base begins with p, *con-* becomes *com-*
when the base begins with r, *con-* becomes *cor-*

For *en-*, when the base begins with l, *en-* becomes *el-*
when the base begins with b, *en-* becomes *em-*
when the base begins with m, *en-* becomes *em-*
when the base begins with p, *en-* becomes *em-*
when the base begins with r, *en-* becomes *er-*

For *in-*, when the base begins with l, *in-* becomes *il-*
when the base begins with b, *in-* becomes *im-*
when the base begins with m, *in-* becomes *im-*
when the base begins with p, *in-* becomes *im-*
when the base begins with r, *in-* becomes *ir-*

For *syn-*, when the base begins with l, *syn-* becomes *syl-*
when the base begins with b, *syn-* becomes *sym-*
when the base begins with m, *syn-* becomes *sym-*
when the base begins with p, *syn-* becomes *sym-*
when the base begins with s, *syn-* becomes *sys-* or *sy-*

For *ob-*, when the base begins with c, *ob-* becomes *oc-*
when the base begins with f, *ob-* becomes *of-*
when the base begins with g, *ob-* becomes *og-*
when the base begins with p, *ob-* becomes *op-*

For *sub-*, when the base begins with c, *sub-* becomes *suc-*
when the base begins with g, *sub-* becomes *sug-*
when the base begins with p, *sub-* becomes *sup-*
when the base begins with r, *sub-* becomes *sur-*

It is not as difficult as it looks. Note how all the prefixes ending in the letter "n" behave in a similar way. Just be aware that if you come across a prefix that you do not immediately recognize, it may be an assimilated form. From now on, the various forms will be listed in the tables of prefixes that you memorize.

This seems like a good place to have a review of the prefixes and suffixes we have learned so far, and to remind ourselves of the basic techniques of building up medical definitions.

Review

CHAPTERS 1–5

PREFIXES

Here are all the prefixes we have come across so far, including any alternative forms that occur because of elision, assimilation, or any other pronunciation change. Remember, prefixes are often prepositions that tell us where something happens (its location or direction), or adverbs that tell us how something happens (its degree, amount or quality), or when. Some prefixes can act as both preposition and adverb; *ante-*, for example, can mean both "before, in front of" in the sense of location, but also in the sense of time.

1. *a-, an-*	without, not, non-
2. *ambi-, ambo-*	both
3. *amphi-, ampho-*	both, on both sides
4. *ante-*	before, in front of
5. *anti-, ant-*	against, opposite
6. *apo-, ap-*	away from
7. *cata-, cat-*	down, complete
8. *circum-*	around
9. *con-, col-, com-, cor-*	together, with
10. *contra-*	opposite, against
11. *de-*	down, downward, away from, from, without, out of
12. *dia-, di-*	through, apart, in a line
13. *dys-*	bad, painful, difficult, abnormal

14. *ec-, ex-*	out, outside
15. *ecto-, ect-*	outside, outer
16. *eiso-, eso-*	inward
17. *en-, el-, em-, er-*	in, inward
18. *endo-, end-*	inside, inner
19. *ento-, ent-*	inside, within
20. *epi-, ep-*	upon, on the surface
21. *eu-*	good, well, normal
22. *extra-, extro-*	outside of, beyond
23. *hemi-*	half
24. *hyper-*	over, above, more than normal
25. *hypo-, hyp-*	below, deficient, less than normal
26. *in-, il-, im-, ir-*	in, into
27. *infra-*	below
28. *inter-*	between
29. *intra-*	within
30. *meso-*	middle
31. *meta-, met-*	after, change, transition
32. *multi-*	many, much
33. *non-*	not
34. *ob-*	toward, in front of, against
35. *para-, par-*	beside, beyond, abnormal
36. *per-*	through
37. *peri-*	around, near
38. *poly-*	many, much
39. *post-*	behind, after
40. *pros-*	toward

41. *re-*	again and again, backward
42. *semi-*	half, partly
43. *sub-, suc-, sug-, sup-, sur-*	below, underneath
44. *super-*	upper, above, beyond
45. *supra-*	above
46. *syn-, syl-, sym-, sys-, sy-*	together, with, concurrent
47. *trans-*	across, through

ADJECTIVE-FORMING SUFFIXES

All of these suffixes form an adjective when added to a base:

1. -aceous	pertaining to, belonging to, having
2. -ad	toward
3. -al, -eal, -ial	pertaining to
4. -alis, -aris	pertaining to
5. -an	pertaining to
6. -ar	pertaining to, having the character of
7. -ary	pertaining to
8. -ate	pertaining to, having, having the shape, to (...)
9. -atic	pertaining to
10. -atory	pertaining to
11. -escent	beginning to be, becoming
12. -etic	pertaining to
13. -form	having the form of, like
14. -iatic	pertaining to a state, pertaining to a process
15. -ible, -ibil-	able to be

16. -ic	pertaining to
17. -ical	pertaining to
18. -ile	pertaining to, able to
19. -ior	pertaining to
20. -ive	pertaining to, tending to
21. -oid	resembling, shaped, like, shaped like
22. -ose	full of, having the quality of
23. -ous	pertaining to, like, full of, having
24. -tic	pertaining to
25. -ual	pertaining to

Note that -ate can also form a verb, the infinitive "to do (something)" when combined with a base.

NOUN-FORMING SUFFIXES

All of these suffixes form a noun when added to a base:

26. -ation	process
27. -duct	duct, channel, tube
28. -ema	condition
29. -esis	condition, abnormal condition, process
30. -ety	condition, state, quality
31. -gen	that which produces
32. -gram	record
33. -graph	instrument used to record
34. -ia	condition of, quality of, state of, act of
35. -iasis	state of, process of, abnormal condition

36. -in	substance
37. -ion	action, condition, act of
38. -itis	inflammation
39. -ity	condition, state, quality
40. -ment	action of, product of
41. -meter	instrument used to measure
42. -oma	tumor, mass
43. -orium	place for
44. -osis	process of, condition of, abnormal condition of
45. -scope	instrument used to examine
46. -sia, -sis	process of, condition of, act of
47. -um	structure, substance
48. -ure	result of, act of
49. -y	condition of, quality of, state of, act of

These two suffixes also form nouns when added to a base, but they form a special type of noun called a diminutive, something that expresses the small size of the thing in question:

50. -cle	small
51. -ula	small

We can also add our compound suffixes here, since they also form nouns when added to a base:

52. -blepsia	condition of sight
53. -cyte	cell
54. -graphy	process of recording
55. -mania	condition of madness, compulsion, obsession

56. -metry	process of measuring
57. -mnesia	condition of memory, memory
58. -opia	condition of sight
59. -opsia	condition of sight
60. -philia	condition of attraction, abnormal craving for
61. -phobia	condition of fear, abnormal fear of
62. -scopy	process of examining with an instrument
63. -verse	to turn, to travel, turned

Note that the suffix -verse can also form an adjective or a verb.

VERB-FORMING SUFFIXES

All of these suffixes form a verb when added to a base:

64. -esce	to begin, to become
65. -ize	to make, to affect

BUILDING UP MEDICAL DEFINITIONS

So, just to review the approach we have used. Suppose that you have broken down your compound term into its individual word parts, prefix(es), suffix(es), base(s), and combining vowel(s); you have accounted for everything in the term and is nothing left over; in what order do you build up your word?

BASE-suffix

The simplest case is just one base and one suffix. Remember, there must be a suffix to complete the sense of the base. Always start with the suffix—this is going to tell you whether your compound term is a noun, adjective, or verb. Then, add in your base, and add in any little words such as "the" or "of" you need to make sense:

frontal (FRONT-al) – pertaining to the front

Sometimes, you might have to add a little more to make a good definition. This is probably the most difficult part because you have to apply a bit of common sense. Here, for example:

steatosis (STEAT-osis) – abnormal condition of fat

Steatosis does mean "abnormal condition of fat," but is it likely that the fat itself is abnormal? A more likely case is that it is a condition in which an abnormal amount of fat is deposited, so you can adjust your definition to reflect this:

steatosis (STEAT-osis) – abnormal condition of fat deposit

This expansion of the term can be difficult at first but, when you have seen a lot more examples, it will become easier.

BASE-CV-suffix

Sometimes, there might be a combining vowel between your base and suffix if the base ends with a consonant and the suffix begins with a consonant. This is to make pronunciation easier. Remember, we always think of the combining vowel as being added to the end of the base, not the beginning of the suffix. Combining vowels are often "o," but they can be the other vowels or the letter "y." Always start with the suffix, then add in your base. Add in any words necessary to make good sense. The combining vowel does not add anything to the definition, but be sure that you can recognize it:

morphotic (MORPH-O-tic) – pertaining to form or shape
collagen (COLL-A-gen) – that which produces glue

BASE-BASE-suffix (AND BASE-CV-BASE-suffix, BASE-BASE-CV-suffix)

Since the combining vowel adds nothing to the definition, we can consider all these cases together. Remember, a combining vowel may occur between bases, or between base and suffix. This is a little more complicated because of the two bases, since sometimes the exact relationship between the two is not explicit. Always start with the suffix, then add the ultimate base (the last base); we can be pretty certain that the suffix completes its sense. Often the suffix applies to both bases and we can just join them with the word "and":

temporoparietal (TEMPOR-O-PARIET-al) – pertaining to the parietal and temporal bones or regions

Sometimes, the suffix cannot apply to both bases; here, for example:

cephalocaudad (CEPHAL-O-CAUD-ad) – toward the tail…the head

Toward the tail and the head at the same time is very unlikely, and we have to supply a bit of common sense to make a useful definition. Remember to add in any words necessary to make good sense:

cephalocaudad (CEPHAL-O-CAUD-ad) – toward the tail from the head

Here is another example, with no combining vowel:

gyrencephalic (GYR-ENCEPHAL-ic) – pertaining to the brain…coil

Again, "pertaining to the brain and a coil" does not seem very likely, and we have to use a bit of common sense to get a good definition.

gyrencephalic (GYR-ENCEPHAL-ic) – pertaining to a brain that has coils, i.e., a brain with many folds

This all becomes easier with practice.

BASE-suffix-suffix (INCLUDING ANY TERMS WITH COMBINING VOWELS)

Occasionally, there may be more than one suffix. Here are three examples we have seen:

gyroidal (GYR-oid-al) – pertaining to shaped like a coil, i.e., spiral

visibility (VIS-ibil-ity) – state of being able to be seen

metricize (METR-ic-ize) – to make pertaining to measurement

Start with the last suffix, add the other suffix, and then add the base. Add in any words necessary to make good sense. It is as if you are making a single suffix out of the two suffixes, and then applying it to your base. This will work for almost all cases, even if there is more than one base. If combining vowels are involved, they do not alter the definition.

prefix-BASE-suffix (INCLUDING ANY TERMS WITH COMBINING VOWELS)

Remember, the prefix adds extra information about the base. Always start with the suffix, then add the prefix, and then add in your base. Add in any words necessary to make good sense.

nonelastic (*non*-ELAST-ic) – pertaining to not flexible

prefix-BASE-BASE-suffix (INCLUDING ANY TERMS WITH COMBINING VOWELS)

We have not come across any compound terms of this type yet. They do exist and we will talk about them when we meet them.

prefix-prefix-BASE-suffix (INCLUDING ANY TERMS WITH COMBINING VOWELS)

The inclusion of more than one prefix in a term is unusual, but does occur occasionally. We have already seen, for example:

antidepressive (*anti-de*-PRESS-ive) – pertaining to against downward pressing, i.e., counteracting feeling of hopelessness

In most cases, always start with the suffix, then add the first prefix, then the second prefix, and then add in your base. Add in any words necessary to make good sense.

RULE-BREAKERS AND ODDITIES

Remember, these are general rules. Like any language, rules get broken sometimes. There will also be oddities. We have already seen, for example:

pupillatonia (PUPILL-*a*-TON-ia) – condition of without tone in the pupil, i.e., the pupil lacks the ability to contract

In this case, a base precedes a *prefix*-BASE-suffix combination. We will talk about other rule-breakers and oddities as we meet them.

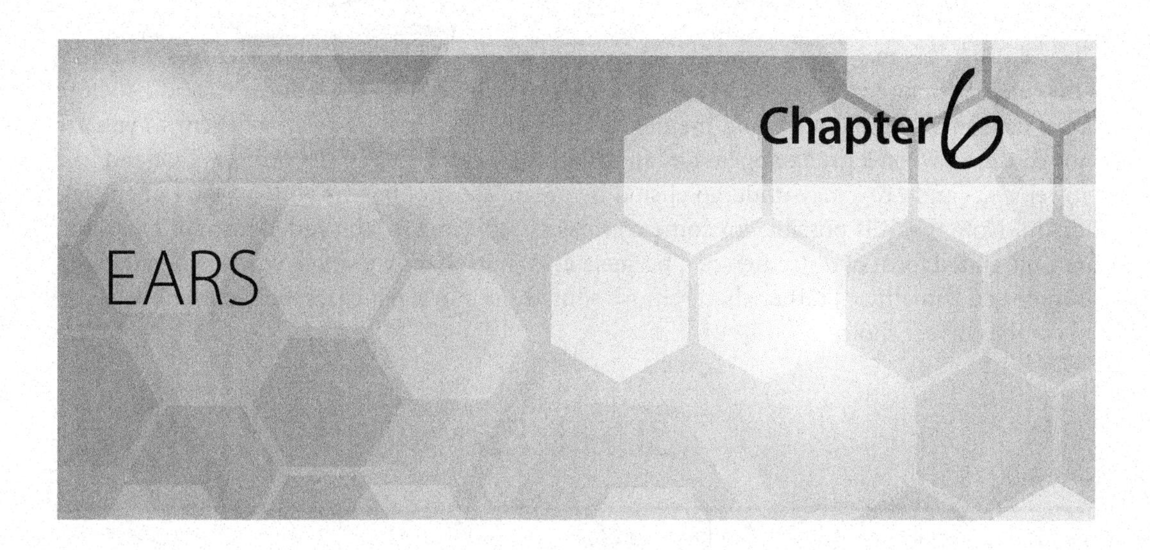

PREFIXES

1. *ana-, an-*	up, upward, again
2. *dis-, dif-, di-*	apart, away from, separation, lack of
3. *enanti-*	opposite
4. *ex-, ef-, e-*	out, outside, from, without
5. *exo-, ex-*	outside, outer, external
6. *in-, il-, im-, ir-*	not
7. *juxta-*	close to
8. *pre-, prae-*	in front of, before
9. *pro-*	in front of, forward
10. *se-*	away, aside
11. *ultra-*	beyond

We have met the prefix *in-*, *il-*, *im-*, *ir-* previously, where it had the meanings "in, into, on, upon." Here, it has a completely unrelated meaning, "not." It follows the same rules of assimilation that we looked at earlier. The prefix *dis* undergoes some changes depending on the first letter of the base that follows; it becomes *dif-* before "f," and *di-* before the letters "b," "d," "g," "l," "m," "n," "r," and "v." The prefix *ex-* also undergoes some changes; as a general rule, *ex-* before vowels, the letter "h," and some consonants, *ef-* before "f," and *e-* before most consonants. Do not try and memorize these changes; just be aware of them so you are not confused when a prefix appears in an unfamiliar form. Two of the prefixes that end in a vowel, *ana-* and *exo-*, may undergo elision before a base that begins with a vowel or the letter "h." Note that it is possible for some confusion between *an-*, the elided form of *ana-*, and *an-*, the elided form of *a-* (remember, because *a-* is in itself only a single vowel, when it elides it must add something, rather than remove something). In most cases, context will help you make the correct choice.

SUFFIXES

1. -able, -abil-	able to be
2. -ac	pertaining to
3. -ance, -ancy	state of
4. -ature	system composed of
5. -culus	small
6. -ent	pertaining to
7. -er	person who (does...), thing that (does...)
8. -fic	causing, making
9. -ician	specialist
10. -ics, -tics	art of, science of, study of
11. -id	pertaining to, having
12. -ine	pertaining to
13. -ism	condition of
14. -ist	person who (does...), specialist
15. -ization	process of making
16. -ory	having the function of

Note that when the suffix -able is combined with another suffix after it, its form changes to -abil-. So, for example, permeable (*per*-ME-able), but permeability (*per*-ME-abil-ity).

BASES

Here are our bases relating to the ear, hearing, and sound:

1. **AUD—to hear, hearing**
   AUDI—to hear, hearing
   AUDIT—to hear, hearing

   audile (AUD-ile) – pertaining to hearing; also, able to hear, i.e., a person who understands better what they hear rather than what they see

   audiometry (AUDI-O-metry) – process of measuring hearing

   auditory (AUDIT-ory) – having the function of hearing

2. **ACOU—hearing, sound**
   ACOUS—hearing, sound

   acoumeter (ACOU-meter) – instrument used to measure hearing

   anacousia (*an*-ACOUS-ia) – condition of not hearing, i.e., deafness

   acousticophobia (ACOUS-tic-O-phobia) – abnormal fear pertaining to sound

Note that acousticophobia is unusual in that it has two suffixes (if we consider -phobia as one of our compound suffixes); also, since the first one ends with a consonant and the second one starts with a consonant, a combining vowel is added to the first suffix. This follows exactly the method we outlined in the last chapter for BASE-suffix-suffix. Start with the final suffix, add the other suffix, and then add the base; add in any words necessary to make good sense, and if combining vowels are involved, they do not alter the definition.

3. **SON—sound**

   asonia (*a*-SON-ia) – condition of without sound, i.e., deafness

   ultrasonography (*ultra*-SON-O-graphy) – process of recording with beyond (normal) sound, i.e., visualizing internal structures using reflected high frequency sound waves

   sonographer (SON-O-GRAPH-er) – person who records with sound, i.e., specialist who uses high-frequency sound waves for diagnosis

   dissonance (*dis*-SON-ance) – state of separation of sound, i.e., a disagreement or discord of sound

4. **AUR—ear**

   dextraural (DEXTR-AUR-al) – pertaining to the right ear

   auriscopy (AUR-I-scopy) – process of examining the ear with an instrument

   auricle (AUR-I-cle) – small ear

Note the combining vowel in auriscopy and in auricle is "i." The term dextraural may refer to a person who prefers to use his or her right ear when answering the phone; a person who prefers to use his or her left ear can be called levoaural or sinistraural (remember, we came across two bases that mean "left"). The term auricle is applied to the part of the outer ear that projects outward from the head, but also to the small, ear-shaped projections found in the heart. We can think of AURICUL- as a base:

5. AURICUL—auricle, outer ear

auricular (AURICUL-ar) – pertaining to the outer ear, pertaining to an auricle

preauricular (*pre*-AURICUL-ar) – pertaining to in front of the outer ear, pertaining to in front of the auricle

auriculocranial (AURICUL-O-CRANI-al) – pertaining to the cranium and the outer ear

auriculoid (AURICUL-oid) – shaped like the outer ear

6. OT—ear

endotitis (*end*-OT-itis) – inflammation of the inner ear

prootic (*pro*-OT-ic) – pertaining to in front of the ear

parotid (*par*-OT-id) – pertaining to beside the ear

Notice that in endotitis, the prefix *endo-* has elided to *end-* because the following base begins with a vowel, and *para-* has elided to *par-* in parotid. The prefix *pro-* does not elide, hence the term prootic, with a slight pause in pronunciation between *pro-* and -OT-ic.

7. PENN—feather, wing
PINN—feather, wing

penniform (PENN-I-form) – like a feather or wing

pinnate (PINN-ate) – pertaining to a feather or wing, having feathers or wings

Note the combining vowel in penniform is "i." Because it is a projecting body part, like a feather or wing, the outer part of the ear is sometimes called the pinna, an alternative to auricle:

PINN—pinna, auricle (the outer ear)

pinnal (PINN-al) – pertaining to the pinna

The pinna is made up from elastic cartilage and overlying skin.

8. CHONDR—granule, cartilage

synchondrosis (*syn*-CHONDR-osis) – condition of (a joint) with cartilage, i.e., a joint where cartilage is the connecting medium between the bones

hypochondriac (*hypo*-CHONDR-I-ac) – pertaining to below the cartilage region (of the breastbone)

hypochondriasis (*hypo*-CHONDR-iasis) – abnormal condition below the cartilage region (of the breastbone), i.e., an abnormal condition affecting the hypochondriac region

The hypochondrium is the part of the abdomen below the cartilaginous breastbone but above the navel. The ancient Greeks believed that this was the place where the bodily humors that caused melancholy resided. When the term hypochondriasis, or hypochondria, first entered medical vocabulary, it was applied to any condition that was believed to be caused by an imbalance of the humors in that region, including disorders of the stomach and digestive system, as well as anxiety and gloominess. Today, the term is used for a condition in which sufferers worry morbidly about having serious illnesses, despite there being no medical evidence of illness.

9. HELIC—spiral, helix

helicine (HELIC-ine) – pertaining to a spiral or helix

helicoid (HELIC-oid) – resembling a spiral or helix

The outer curled edge of the auricle (or pinna) is termed the helix; the inner rim of the edge is termed the antihelix.

10. FOSS—ditch, trench, to dig

efossion (*e*-FOSS-ion) – action of removal by digging, i.e., digging out or up

In anatomy, a pit, a trenchlike depression, or a hollow in the surface of a structure in the body is called a fossa:

FOSS—fossa

fossula (FOSS-ula) – a little fossa, i.e., a small depression or hollow

In the ear, the triangular fossa is a shallow depression between two parts of the antihelix.

11. SCAPH—boat shaped

scaphocephalism (SCAPH-O-CEPHAL-ism) – condition of the head being boat shaped, i.e., a condition in which the cranial bones fuse abnormally, resulting in a long narrow head (like an inverted boat)

scaphoid (SCAPH-oid) – shaped like a boat

In the ear, the scaphoid fossa is a boat-shaped groove inside the helix.

12. TUBER—swelling, nodule

tubercle (TUBER-cle) - small swelling

In the ear, the tubercle is a small bump on the helix, sometimes called Darwin's tubercle because he mentions it in his famous work, *Descent of Man.* We can think of TUBERCUL- as a base:

13. TUBERCUL—tubercle, small swelling or nodule

tuberculitis (TUBERCUL-itis) - inflammation of any tubercle

tuberculosis (TUBERCUL-osis) - abnormal condition of the tubercles

More specifically, tuberculosis is a disease caused by the bacterium *Mycobacterium tuberculosis*, often located in the lungs.

14. CONCH—seashell, spiral shell

conchate (CONCH-ate) - pertaining to a seashell

conchiform (CONCH-I-form) - having the form of a spiral shell

In anatomy, a concha (plural conchae) is a structure similar in shape to a seashell. Note the combining vowel in conchiform is "i." In the ear, the concha is an area of the auricle (or pinna) between helix and antihelix. In the nose, the conchae are long, thin, spongy bones that are curved like a seashell:

CONCH—concha

conchitis (CONCH-itis) - inflammation of a concha

conchoscope (CONCH-O-scope) - an instrument used to examine the conchae

Sometimes, the conchae are called turbinates:

15. TURBIN—cone shaped, spiraled

turbinate (TURBIN-ate) - having cone-shaped (features)

turbinated (TURBIN-ated) - composed of spiraled (parts)

turbinectomy (TURBIN-ectomy) - surgical removal of a turbinated (bone)

16. MAST—breast

amastia (*a*-MAST-ia) - condition of without breasts

mastoid (MAST-oid) - resembling a breast

Just behind the outer ear, there is a bony projection from the temporal bone; because this rounded bone was thought to resemble a breast, it was termed the mastoid process (see below for the term process). We can think of MASTOID- as a base:

17. MASTOID—mastoid process

mastoiditis (MASTOID-itis) – inflammation of the mastoid process

premastoidal (*pre*-MASTOID-al) – pertaining to in front of the mastoid process

18. CED—to go, to be in motion
CESS—to go, to be in motion

antecedent (*ante*-CED-ent) – pertaining to before going, i.e., going before

processive (*pro*-CESS-ive) – tending to forward moving

secession (*se*-CESS-ion) – act of away moving, i.e., a withdrawal

In anatomy, processes (singular process, *pro*-CESS, literally "to go forward" or "in front of") are bony projections that provide attachment points for muscles and ligaments. Just below the ear, the temporal styloid process, a slender and pointed piece of bone, projects down and forward from the temporal bone:

19. STYL—column, pillar

styloid (STYL-oid) – resembling a column

styliform (STYL-I-form) – having the form of a column

Note the combining vowel in styliform is "i." We can think of STYLOID- as a base:

20. STYL—styloid process
STYLOID—styloid process

stylomastoidal (STYL-O-MASTOID-al) – pertaining to the mastoid and styloid processes (of the temporal bone)

styloiditis (STYLOID-itis) – inflammation of a styloid process

Note that there are also styloid processes associated with bones other than the temporal bone.

21. ME—to go, to pass, to travel

permeation (*per*-ME-ation) – process of through passage, i.e., process of passing through something

permeable (*per*-ME-able) – tending to (allow) through passage, i.e., permitting passage of substances

impermeable (*im-per*-ME-able) – tending to not (allow) through passage, i.e., not permitting passages of substances

Notice that impermeable is unusual in that it has two prefixes. We can use the same method we used previously for terms of this sort (*prefix-prefix*-BASE-suffix)—start with the suffix, then add the first prefix, then the second prefix, and then add in your base. Remember, the prefix *in-* becomes *im-* when the following base begins with the letter "p," due to the process of assimilation. In anatomy, the term meatus (literally, "something that is traveled") is applied to a bodily passage or channel, especially the external opening of a canal:

22. MEAT—opening, passageway, meatus

meatal (MEAT-al) – pertaining to an opening, pertaining to a meatus

meatoscopy (MEAT-O-scopy) – process of examining a meatus with an instrument

meatometry (MEAT-O-metry) – process of measuring a meatus

In the ear, the canal leading from the outer ear to the middle ear is called the external auditory meatus. Just in front of it, on the external ear, is a triangular piece of cartilage, called the tragus. It gets its name from the Greek word for goat, *tragos*, since this part of the ear often becomes hairy (especially in old age), just like a goat's beard. The only other medical terms associated with *tragos* that you may come across are tragomaschalia, a condition of having armpits that smell like a goat, tragopodia, a condition of the feet and knees like a goat (knock knees), and tragophonia, a condition of the voice that makes it sound like a bleating goat.

23. TYMPAN—drum, stretched membrane

tympanal (TYMPAN-al) – pertaining to a drum

tympanism (TYMPAN-ism) – condition of (being like) a drum, i.e., a condition in which the abdomen is stretched like a drum due to gas in the intestinal cavity

In the ear, the membrane that separates the outer ear from the middle ear is termed the tympanic membrane (eardrum), while the tympanic cavity is a small chamber surrounding the bones of the middle ear:

TYMPAN—tympanic membrane, tympanic cavity

tympanotemporal (TYMPAN-O-TEMPOR-al) – pertaining to the tympanic cavity and the temporal region or bone

tympanitis (TYMPAN-itis) – inflammation of the tympanic membrane

tympanometry (TYMPAN-O-metry) – process of measuring (movement of) the tympanic membrane

tympanogenous (TYMPAN-O-GEN-ous) – pertaining to production by the tympanic cavity, i.e., originating in the tympanic cavity

24. MYRING—tympanic membrane

myringitis (MYRING-itis) – inflammation of the tympanic membrane

myringoscope (MYRING-O-scope) instrument used to examine the tympanic membrane

25. OSS—bone
OSSE—bone

ossature (OSS-ature) – system composed of bones, i.e., a skeletal framework

ossicle (OSS-I-cle) – small bone

osseous (OSSE-ous) – pertaining to bone

In the ear, there are three ossicles in the tympanic cavity, the malleus (hammer), incus (anvil), and stapes (stirrup). They got their names because they resemble the shapes of a hammer and anvil, and a stirrup; malleus and incus are both Latin words, but the word stapes is a fairly modern invention (the ancient Greeks and Romans did not use stirrups when riding). The auditory ossicles are responsible for transmitting vibrations from the tympanic membrane to the inner ear.

26. LABYRINTH—labyrinth, maze

labyrinthine (LABYRINTH-ine) – pertaining to a labyrinth

In Greek mythology, the labyrinth was a vast underground maze created for King Minos on the island of Crete. The Minotaur—part bull, part man—was confined to its depths, feasting on the flesh of the seven youths and seven maidens that were sent every year from Athens to Minos as recompense for an old crime. The hero Theseus entered the labyrinth, unwinding a ball of thread as he went, killed the Minotaur, and was able to find his way out by following the thread back to the entrance. In anatomy, several structures that are characterized by numerous interconnecting chambers and canals are termed labyrinths. The inner ear, composed of the vestibule, semicircular ducts, and cochlea, is termed a labyrinth:

LABYRINTH—inner ear

labyrinthitis (LABYRINTH-itis) – inflammation of the inner ear

27. VESTIBUL—vestibule, entrance

vestibulate (VESTIBUL-ate) – having a vestibule

vestibular (VESTIBUL-ar) – pertaining to a vestibule

In anatomy, a vestibule (or, vestibulum) is a small entrance to a canal. In the ear, the vestibule is the entrance to the inner ear.

28. COCHLE—snail shell, spiral shell

cochleous (COCHLE-ous) – like a snail shell

cochleate (COCHLE-ate) – pertaining to a snail shell

In the inner ear, the cochlea is a spiral-shaped canal surrounding a core of spongy bone:

COCHLE—cochlea

cochlear (COCHLE-ar) – pertaining to the cochlea

cochleitis (COCHLE-itis) – inflammation of the cochlea

vestibulocochlear (VESTIBUL-O-COCHLE-ar) – pertaining to the vestibule and cochlea

29. CANAL—channel

canaliform (CANAL-I-form) – having the form of a channel

canaliculus (CANAL-I-culus) – a small channel, a canaliculus

In anatomy, a canal is a channel or duct, usually a tubular structure. In the ear, the semicircular canals are bony structures housing the semicircular ducts that play a vital role in balancing the body. Note the combining vowel in both canaliform and canaliculus is "i." A canaliculus is a small canal or channel in the body. The suffix -culus is another of the diminutive forming suffixes such as -cle, and -ula. We can think of CANALICUL- as a base:

30. CANALICUL—canaliculus, small channel

canalicular (CANALICUL-ar) – pertaining to a canaliculus

canaliculization (CANALICUL-ization) – process of making canaliculi (plural of canaliculus), or small channels, in a tissue

31. AMPULL—flask, bottle

ampulliform (AMPULL-I-form) – having the form of a flask or bottle

Note the combining vowel in ampulliform is "i." In anatomy, an ampulla is a flask-shaped enlargement of a canal or duct:

AMPULL—ampulla

ampullitis (AMPULL-itis) – inflammation of an ampulla

juxtaampullary (*juxta*-AMPULL-ary) – pertaining to close to an ampulla

ampullula (AMPULL-ula) – small ampulla

In the ear, each of the semicircular canals has an ampulla, a flask-shaped enlargement, at one end. Remember, some prefixes that end in a vowel do not elide, that is they do not lose their final vowel when they are joined to a base that begins with a vowel. The prefix *juxta-* does not elide, so here we get the slightly odd looking term juxtaampullary. You might come across it in its hyphenated form juxta-ampullary; both forms are correct. Using a hyphen occurs most often when the prefix ends in the same vowel that the base begins with, as we have here.

SOME MORE THINGS TO LEARN

Here are some bases to learn that relate to pain, disease, and treatment:

32. ALG—pain

algogenesis (ALG-O-GEN-esis) – process of producing pain

otalgia (OT-ALG-ia) – condition of pain in the ear, i.e., earache

algophobia (ALG-O-phobia) – abnormal fear of pain

33. ALGES—pain sensation

analgesic (*an*-ALGES-ic) – pertaining to without pain sensation, i.e., something that alleviates pain

algesimetry (ALGES-I-metry) – process of measuring pain sensation

hyperalgesia (*hyper*-ALGES-ia) – condition of more than normal pain sensation

Note the combining vowel in algesimetry is "i."

34. AGR—pain, painful seizure

cephalagra (CEPHAL-AGRa) – pain in the head

ophthalmagra (OPHTHALM-AGRa) – pain in the eyes

The base AGR- is unusual in that you will probably never come across it other than in the combination AGRa, which is actually an unmodified Greek noun and not a true BASE-suffix combination. It is probably better to think of it only as one of the compound suffixes.

35. ODYN—pain

otodynia (OT-ODYN-ia) – condition of pain in the ear, i.e., earache

anodynia (*an*-ODYN-ia) – condition of (being) without pain

cephalodynic (CEPHAL-ODYN-ic) – pertaining to pain in the head

36. DOL—pain
DOLOR—pain

indolent (*in*-DOL-ent) – pertaining to not painful, i.e., causing little pain

dolorific (DOLOR-I-fic) – causing pain

Note the combining vowel in dolorific is "i."

37. NOS—disease, sickness

nosogenic (NOS-O-GEN-ic) – pertaining to producing disease

gynenosia (GYN-E-NOS-ia) – condition of disease that (affects) women (mostly)

nosometry (NOS-O-metry) – process of measuring disease, i.e., the quantification of the extent of a disease in a population

Note the combining vowel in gynenosia is "e."

38. MORB—disease

morbid (MORB-id) – pertaining to disease

morbigenous (MORB-I-GEN-ous) – pertaining to the production of disease

Note the combining vowel in morbigenous is "i."

39. PATH—disease, suffering, feeling

andropathy (ANDR-O-PATH-y) – state of a disease that (affects) men (mostly)

enantiopathic (*enanti*-O-PATH-ic) – pertaining to opposite feelings

exopathic (*exo*-PATH-ic) – pertaining to an external disease, i.e., a disease originating outside the body

40. AESTHE—to feel, sensation, feeling
ESTHE—to feel, sensation, feeling

anaesthetic (*an*-AESTHE-tic) – pertaining to the condition of without sensation

acouesthesia (ACOU-ESTHE-sia) – condition of sensation of sound, i.e., the sense of hearing

hyperphotesthesia (*hyper*-PHOT-ESTHE-sia) – condition of more than normal sensation to light

anacatesthesia (*ana-cat*-ESTHE-sia) – condition of up down sensation, i.e., a sensation of hovering

The term anacatesthesia is unusual in that it has two prefixes, but we can use the same method to build up the term that we described earlier. Start with the suffix, then add the first prefix, then the second prefix, and then add in your base; add in any words necessary to make good sense. Note that the prefix *cata-* has undergone elision to *cat-* because the following base begins with a vowel. Hyperphotesthesia is the first term we have come across that has the format *prefix*-BASE-BASE-suffix. How do we go about building up our medical term? We know that we should start with the suffix, since this is going to tell us whether the compound term is a noun, adjective, or verb. Here, the suffix -sia tells us we are dealing with a noun, a "condition." With only one base, we would know that the prefix is adding more information about it, and we would move to it next, but here, how do we know which base, or bases, the prefix is modifying? Unfortunately, there is no rule, and we have to use some common sense. If we forget about the prefix for the moment and concentrate on the relationship between the bases and the suffix, using the method we have seen earlier, the suffix could be applying to ESTHE- only, or both PHOT- and ESTHE- (almost impossible for it to be applying to PHOT- only because a suffix applies at least to the base closest to it). Therefore, our choices are "condition of sensation to light" and "condition of sensation and light." The second option really does not make sense, so let us assume that we are talking about a condition of sensation to light. Now looking at our prefix, *hyper-* ("more than normal"), is "condition of sensation to more than normal light" or "condition of more than normal sensation to light" more likely? It is not an obvious choice, since both make some sense. However, if we think about it, surely everyone would experience a sensation to more than normal light and this would not be considered a condition worthy of note. On the other hand, being more sensitive to light than normal would be considered a notable condition, and this gives us our answer. Not easy, but not impossible to build up our medical term if you apply some common sense. We will look closely at other *prefix*-BASE-BASE-suffix type terms as we meet them.

41. THERAP—to provide treatment, treatment
THERAPEUT—treatment

therapist (THERAP-ist) – specialist who provides treatment
therapeutic (THERAPEUT-ic) – pertaining to treatment
therapeutician (THERAPEUT-ician) – specialist who provides treatment

42. IATR—physician, medical treatment

psychiatry (PSYCH-IATR-y) – act of medical treatment of the mind
psychiatrics (PSYCH-IATR-ics) – art of medical treatment of the mind
dermiatric (DERM-IATR-ic) – pertaining to the medical treatment of skin
iatrophobia (IATR-O-phobia) – abnormal fear of physicians

Here are some more compound suffixes, using these new bases and some bases we learned previously. Remember, it is helpful to memorize all the compound suffixes because they occur so regularly, but you can also always build them up from their individual base and suffix parts.

1. -agra	pain, painful seizure
2. -algesia	sensation of pain
3. -algia	painful condition
4. -acousia	condition of hearing
5. -esthesia	condition of sensation
6. -genesis	production
7. -genic	producing, produced
8. -genous	producing, produced
9. -iatrics, -iatry	medical treatment
10. -nosia	disease
11. -odynia	painful condition
12. -pathia, -pathy	disease, treatment of disease
13. -therapia, -therapy	treatment

Most of these compound suffixes are noun-forming suffixes, except for -genic and -genous, which are adjective-forming suffixes.

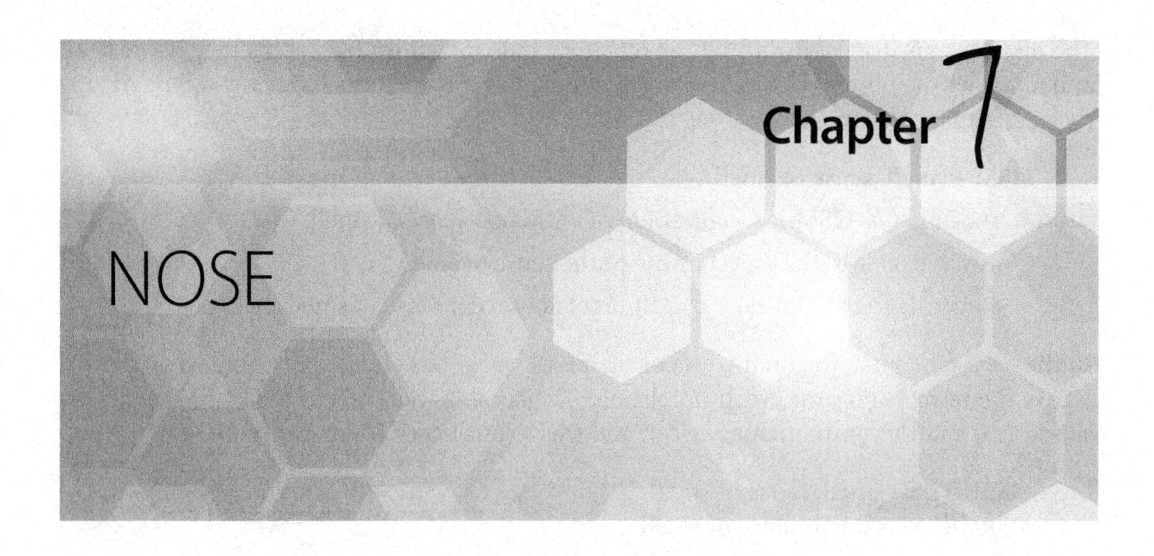

PREFIXES

1. *mal-*	bad, inadequate

SUFFIXES

1. -ant	pertaining to
2. -or	person who (does...), thing that (does...)
3. -plasm	formed substance, growth
4. -tome	instrument used to cut

BASES

1. OLFACT—smell, sense of smell

olfactor (OLFACT-or) – thing that has a sense of smell, i.e., nose

olfaction (OLFACT-ion) – the act of smelling

olfactory (OLFACT-ory) – having the function of smelling

The olfactory apparatus, including the olfactory bulb, olfactory tract, olfactory nerve cells, and olfactory membranes, is the sensory unit that gets information about any odor carrying molecules that enter the nose.

2. **OSM—smell, sense of smell**

    anosmia (*an*-OSM-ia) – condition of without a sense of smell

    osmatic (OSM-atic) – pertaining to the sense of smell

    parosmia (*par*-OSM-ia) – condition of abnormal sense of smell

In the term parosmia, the final vowel of the prefix *para-* has elided, but you may also come across the term paraosmia, with no elision. The combination of the base OSM- with the suffix -ia is a fairly common one; we can add this to our list of compound suffixes.

3. **OSPHRES—smell, sense of smell**
    OSPHRESI—smell, sense of smell

    hyperosphresia (*hyper*-OSPHRES-ia) – condition of more than normal sense of smell

    osphresiophobia (OSPHRESI-O-phobia) – abnormal fear of (bad) smells

4. **ODOR—odor, smell**

    malodorous (*mal*-ODOR-ous) – full of bad odor

    deodorant (*de*-ODOR-ant) – pertaining to without odor

    odorimetry (ODOR-I-metry) – process of measuring odor

Note the combining vowel in odorimetry is "i."

5. **NAS—nose**

    nasal (NAS-al) – pertaining to the nose

    nasociliary (NAS-O-CILI-ary) – pertaining to the eyelids and nose

    nasoscope (NAS-O-scope) – instrument used to examine the nose

6. **RHIN—nose**
    -RRHIN—nose

    rhinaesthesia (RHIN-AESTHE-sia) – condition of sensation in the nose, i.e., sense of smell

    rhinalgia (RHIN-algia) – painful condition of the nose

    rhinotome (RHIN-O-tome) – instrument used to cut the nose

    rhinoplasm (RHIN-O-plasm) – formed substance for the nose, i.e., repair material for reconstruction of the nose, although the term is most often seen as an outdated alternative to rhinoplasty

The form -RRHIN- only occurs in the middle of a term, never at the beginning.

7. NAR—nostril

internarial (*inter*-NAR-ial) – pertaining to between the nostrils
nariform (NAR-I-form) – having the form of nostrils

Note the combining vowel in nariform is "i." The nares are the external openings, or nostrils, of the nose; each flared part of the nostril, at the outer edge of the nose, is called an ala (plural alae):

8. AL—wing

alar (AL-ar) – pertaining to a wing or winged structure
alinasal (AL-I-NAS-al) – pertaining to the nose wings

Note the combining vowel in alinasal is "i." In anatomy, the term ala can be applied to any winglike, or wing-shaped, part of a structure.

9. SEPT—(i) dividing wall: (ii) seven

septal (SEPT-al) – pertaining to a dividing wall

In anatomy, a dividing wall between two cavities or areas of soft tissue is called a septum. In the nose, the nasal septum is a wall of cartilage that divides the nasal cavity into two sides:

SEPT—septum

septate (SEPT-ate) – having a septum
eseptate (*e*-SEPT-ate) – being without a septum
septonasal (SEPT-O-NAS-al) – pertaining to the nasal septum

We will look at the meaning "seven" in another chapter.

10. MUC—mucus

mucous (MUC-ous) – pertaining to mucus
mucocutaneous (MUC-O-CUTANE-ous) – pertaining to the skin and mucous membrane

The nasal cavity is lined with membranes that produce mucus, a secretion that consists of the protein mucin, various cells, and inorganic salts. Mucus prevents the underlying tissues from drying out and, with the help of the hairs in the nostrils, it traps inhaled particles such as dust, smoke, and pollen, along with bacteria and fungal spores, and prevents them from traveling to the lungs. In anatomy, a mucus-producing membrane that lines certain bodily structures is termed a mucosa. We can think of MUCOS- as a base:

11. MUCOS—mucosa, mucous membrane

mucosal (MUCOS-al) – pertaining to a mucosa

Profuse discharge of mucus from the nose is called coryza. Here are two more bases that mean mucus, although they are rarely used about mucus in the nasal cavity:

12. BLENN—mucus

blennophthalmia (BLENN-OPHTHALM-ia) – condition of the eyes (caused by) mucus, i.e., usually an inflammation of the conjunctiva

blennogenic (BLENN-O-genic) – producing mucus

13. MYX—mucus

myxoid (MYX-oid) – resembling mucus

myxocyte (MYX-O-cyte) – cell in mucus (producing tissue)

The abnormal amount of mucus that is produced by an inflamed respiratory system (breathing system) is generally called phlegm, especially if it is voided through the mouth:

14. PHLEGM—phlegm, inflammation

phlegmasia (PHLEGM-A-sia) – condition of inflammation

phlegmy (PHLEGM-y) – (having the) quality of phlegm

Note the combining vowel in phlegmasia is "a." Ancient Greek medical theory believed that the body was composed of four humors, or fluids. Phlegm was one of the four, the others being yellow bile, black bile, and blood, although sometimes the two biles were classed as one and a watery substance, hydrops, made up the fourth. When the four humors were in balance and properly mixed, the body was healthy; imbalance, or the separation of one humor from the rest, caused sickness.

15. SIN—curve, cavity

sinuate (SIN-U-ate) – having a curved (shape)

Note the combining vowel in sinuate is "u." In anatomy, a sinus is usually a hollow cavity, or channel leading to a cavity. Four pairs of sinuses are related to the nose; they are called the paranasal sinuses. We can think of SINUS- as a base:

16. SIN—sinus
SINUS—sinus

perisinuous (*peri*-SIN-U-ous) – pertaining to around a sinus

sinusitis (SINUS-itis) – inflammation of the sinuses

rhinosinusopathia (RHIN-O-SINUS-O-pathia) – disease of the sinuses and nose

Note the combining vowel in perisinuous is "u."

SOME MORE THINGS TO LEARN

Here are some more bases to learn. We will see that they all have compound suffixes associated with them.

17. PLAS—to form, to mold
PLAST—to form, to mold

hyperplasia (*hyper*-PLAS-ia) – condition of more than normal formation (of tissue)

anaplasty (*ana*-PLAST-y) – act of again formation, i.e., restoring or reforming body parts, reconstructive surgery

rhinoplasty (RHIN-O-PLAST-y) – act of forming the nose, i.e., reconstructive surgery of the nose

theleplasty (THEL-E-PLAST-y) – act of forming the nipple, i.e., reconstructive surgery of the nipple

Note the combining vowel in theleplasty is "e"; sometimes, you might see this term with "y" as the combining vowel—thelyplasty.

18. CENTE—to puncture

ophthalmocentesis (OPHTHALM-O-CENTE-sis) – process of puncturing the eye, i.e., process of puncturing the eye in order to drain it

tympanocentesis (TYMPAN-O-CENTE-sis) – process of puncturing the tympanic membrane, i.e., process of puncturing the tympanic membrane in order to drain the ear

craniocentesis (CRANI-O-CENTE-sis) – process of puncturing the cranium, i.e., process of puncturing the cranium to reduce the size of an enlarged fetal head to aid delivery

You will probably only ever come across the base CENTE- in the combination CENTE- and the suffix -sis, but this compound suffix -centesis is fairly widespread.

19. TOM—to cut, to slice, section

tomography (TOM-O-graphy) – process of recording sections (of the body)

tomophopbia (TOM-O-phobia) – abnormal fear of being cut, i.e., fear of surgical operations

ototomy (OT-O-TOM-y) – act of cutting the ear, i.e., dissection of the ear

If we add the suffix -e (which has no meaning) to this base, we get the suffix -tome meaning "instrument used to cut." Since it really is a base and suffix combined, we will add it to our list of compound suffixes, along with -verse and -cyte.

20. ECTOM—to cut out, to cut away

adipectomy (ADIP-ECTOM-y) – act of cutting out fat

blepharectomy (BLEPHAR-ECTOM-y) – act of cutting away the eyelid

craniectomy (CRANI-ECTOM-y) – act of cutting out (part of) the cranium

ECTOM- is actually a compound of TOM- with the prefix *ec-* meaning "out," but it has also become used as a base in its own right.

21. STOM—mouth, opening
STOMAT—mouth, opening

dacryocystostomy (DACRY-O-CYST-O-STOM-y) – act of (creating) an opening in the sac related to tears, i.e., act of creating an opening in the lacrimal sac

anastomosis (*ana*-STOM-osis) – process of up-opening, i.e., process of opening up, creation of an opening between two normally separate structures in order to join them

stomatodynia (STOMAT-odynia) – painful condition of the mouth

stomatitis (STOMAT-itis) – inflammation of the mouth

The term dacryocystostomy is the first term we have come across that has three bases (BASE-BASE-BASE-suffix), but we can begin by approaching it the same way we did for terms with two bases (BASE-BASE-suffix). Remember, the combining vowels add nothing to the sense, so we can ignore them. Start with the suffix, then add in the base that is closest to it, since we can be pretty certain that the suffix completes its sense. Remember to add in any words necessary to make good sense. So, we have "act of (creating) an opening." With terms of two bases, we then considered whether the suffix also applied to the base that was next closest, and whether we could just join the two bases with the word "and." Here, that would give us "act of (creating) an opening and the sac," which does not make a great deal of sense. In this instance, we might suspect that any extra bases are going to tell us how or where we are creating an opening. Since "act of (creating) an opening with a sac" seems unlikely, we might consider the alternative "act of (creating) an opening in the sac," and this certainly seems to make reasonable sense. We are then left with a base that means tears. Again, joining this base with the word "and" does not seem right, since the "act of (creating) an opening in the sac and tears" is nonsense. However, if we use a little common sense, we can come up with the "act of (creating) an opening in the sac related to tears," which does indeed make sense, especially as we have seen earlier that the "sac related to tears" is the lacrimal sac. So, as terms get longer, we do have to think more closely about how bases relate to one another, but the process of building up the definition is not an impossible one. Let us make dacryocystostomy even longer:

conjunctivodacryocystostomy (CONJUNCTIV-O-DACRY-O-CYST-O-STOM-y)

Use the same approach as before, beginning with the suffix and the base closest to it, then working backward through the bases, ignoring combining vowels. You might end up with the definition "act of (creating) an opening in the sac related to tears and the conjunctiva." This makes some sense, but seems to imply we are making an opening in two places. Since openings generally begin at one place and end at another, an even more sensible definition is "act of (creating) an opening **between** the sac related to tears and the conjunctiva," and this is, in fact, the definition of conjunctivodacryocystostomy. If you found this process a little intimidating, do not worry, it all comes with practice, and the more terms you look at, the more patterns you will see emerging. Any term using STOM-y, the "act of (creating) an opening," for example, generally involves either one other base that situates the opening in one particular location, or two other bases that situate the opening as occurring between one location and another. So when you see the term dacryocystorhinostomy, you will quite quickly recognize the format and the meaning "act of (creating) an opening between the nose and sac related to tears."

In anatomy, a stoma (plural stomas or stomata) is an opening or pore in the body, including artificial openings.

STOM—stoma

stomal (STOM-al) – pertaining to a stoma

22. CLEI—to close
CLEIST—closed

corecleisis (CORE-CLEI-sis) – condition of closure of the pupil of the eye

cleistophobia (CLEIST-O-phobia) – abnormal fear of closed (spaces)

23. CLAS—to break, fragment

aclasia (*a*-CLAS-ia) – condition of without a break, i.e., continuity between normal and abnormal body tissues

aclassis (*a*-CLAS-sis) – condition of without a break, i.e., continuity between normal and abnormal body tissues

histoclastic (HIST-O-CLAS-tic) – pertaining to breaking (down) of tissue

In the term aclassis, a base ending with "s" is followed by a suffix beginning with "s." In this case, both of the letters "s" are retained, but this is quite unusual. More commonly, the final "s" of the base gets dropped. For example:

trichoclasis (TRICH-O-CLA(S)-sis) – condition of breakage of the hair

24. DE—to bind

syndesis (*syn*-DE-sis) – condition of together binding, i.e., fusion

25. PEX—to fasten, to fix

adipopexia (ADIP-O-PEX-ia) – state of fixing fat (in the body), i.e., state of fat storage

retinopexy (RETIN-O-PEX-y) – act of fastening the retina, i.e., act of repair of detached retina

Another term for fixing fat in the body is lipopexis. It looks as if the suffix in this term is -is, but this is not the case. We saw above with trichoclasis that, when two "s" letters come together, one at the end of the base, the other at the beginning of the suffix, the "s" from the base often gets dropped. Here we are concerned with the letter "x" at the end of the base, but the sound of this letter in ancient Greek was always "ks." The sound of what we have is LIP-O-PEKS-sis and the final "s" sound of -PEKS does indeed get dropped. This still leaves us with a "ks" combination which is rendered by the letter "x." The suffix, then, in this term is actually -sis, it is just hidden.

26. LY—to loosen, dissolving

lipolysis (LIP-O-LY-sis) – process of dissolving fat, i.e., process of splitting up, or decomposition, of fat

dermatolysis (DERMAT-O-LY-sis) – process of loosening of the skin

dialysis (*dia*-LY-sis) – process of apart dissolving, i.e., process of dissolving, filtration, or separation

27. CLY—to wash

clysis (CLY-sis) – process of washing, i.e., process of an infusion of fluid

28. TRIB—to rub, to crush
TRIPS—to rub, to crush

tribometer (TRIB-O-meter) – instrument used to measure rubbing (friction)

cephalotripsy (CEPHAL-O-TRIPS-y) – act of crushing the head, i.e., crushing the head of a fetus to effect delivery

Here are some compound suffixes using these new bases. They can all relate to medical procedures, as well as other less specific processes. Remember, it is helpful to memorize all the compound suffixes because they occur so regularly, but you can also always build them up from their individual base and suffix parts.

1. -centesis	surgical puncturing, puncturing
2. -clasia, -clasis	surgical fracture, breaking, rupture
3. -cleisis	surgical closure, closure
4. -clysis	therapeutic infusion of liquid, irrigation
5. -desis	surgical fusion, binding
6. -dialysis	surgical dissolving, surgical separation, filtration
7. -ectomy	surgical removal, removal
8. -lysis	surgical dissolving, surgical separation, loosening
9. -pexis, -pexy	surgical fastening, fixing
10. -plasia, -plasty	surgical reshaping, formation
11. -stomy	making a surgical opening, making an opening
12. -tripsy	surgical crushing, crushing
13. -tomy	surgical cutting, cutting

In addition, here is the compound suffix we mentioned earlier:

14. -osmia	condition of sense of smell

The final two new bases for this chapter do have compound suffixes of a sort associated with them, but they also have a couple of unusual features:

29. RHAPH—to stitch, to suture
-RRHAPH—to stitch, to suture

blepharorrhaphy (BLEPHAR-O-RRHAPH-y) – act of suturing the eyelid
rhinorrhaphy (RNIN-O-RRHAPH-y) – act of suturing the nose

The form -RRHAPH- only occurs in the middle of a term, never at the beginning. The base RHAPH- rarely appears in medical terminology; you will probably only ever come across it in the term rhaphe, the ridge that forms a seam between two structures.

30. RHE—to flow
-RRH—to flow

rheoencephalography (RHE-O-ENCEPHAL-O-graphy) – process of recording brain (blood) flow

cryptorrhetic (CRYPT-O-RRH-etic) – pertaining to flow that is hidden, i.e., pertaining to secreting internally

catarrhal (*cata*-RRH-al) – pertaining to down flow, i.e., pertaining to catarrh, the increased flow of mucus

The form -RRH- only occurs in the middle or end of a term, never at the beginning.

Here is the first unusual feature of these bases, their compound suffixes:

15. -rrhage	excessive flow, excessive discharge
16. -rrhagia	excessive flow, excessive discharge
17. -rrhaphy	surgical suture
18. -rrhea	flow, discharge
19. -rrhexis	rupture

The compound -rrhaphy is formed quite regularly from the modified base -RRHAPH- and the suffix -y. The others are much closer to their original Greek forms and do not use any of our regular suffixes. They are not true compound suffixes in the way we have described them so far, but they are fairly common and you should memorize them. You will not be able to build them up from their individual base and suffix parts.

The second unusual feature is the "rrh," the form that appears in the middle of terms; we also saw it associated with the base RHIN-, where we see the form -RRHIN- in the middle of words, and in the term CIRRH-osis. We will see it with other bases later. It looks quite strange to users of the English language. It is not necessary to know why it comes about, just be sure to recognize it and know what bases it is associated with. However, for those who are interested, it occurs because of certain peculiarities of the Greek language from which the relevant bases are derived. Ancient Greek had no equivalent of our letter "h." Vowels at the beginning of the word could be pronounced with a release of breath, a process called aspiration, or not. It is like the difference between the pronunciation of "hour" and "our," but Greek indicated the difference with a mark placed over the vowel. The Greek equivalent of the letter "r" was also aspirated whenever it was at the beginning of a word, so something like "r-h," the sound that we get at the beginning of the word rhythm. If any sort of prefix that ended in a vowel was added in front of such a word, the letter "r" was duplicated, the second "r" being aspirated, the first one not, giving us "rrh." This is just a rule of ancient Greek pronunciation that we have to accept.

In general, the practice has been to reflect the ancient rules in the spelling of medical terminology, even if we do not really attempt to pronounce it, hence the "rrh" combination in the middle of words. However, there is some inconsistency, and increasingly you might see "rh" replacing the "rrh" form, as in, for example, cirhosis, rhinorhaphy, and cryptorhetic.

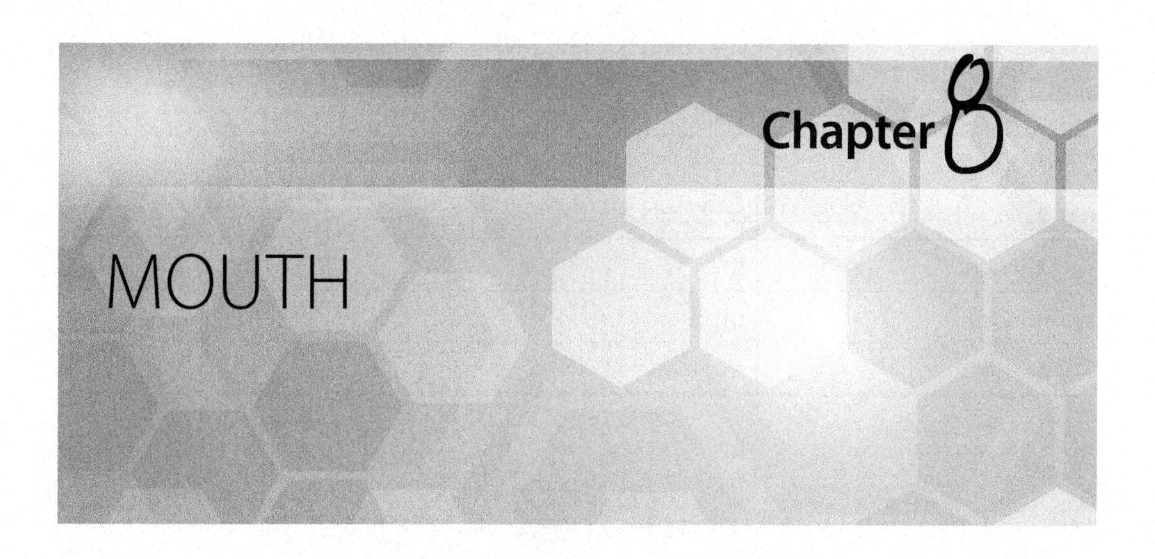

PREFIXES

1. *ab-, a-*	away from
2. *ad-, ac-, af-* etc.	toward, near
3. *retro-*	behind, backward

The prefix *ab-* undergoes some changes depending on the first letter of the base that follows; as a general rule, *ab-* before vowels and the letter "h," *a-* before consonants. Note that there is the possibility of confusion with the prefix *a-/an-*. The prefix *ad-* undergoes assimilation before certain consonants—remember, we said that sometimes the final consonant of a prefix changes to something closer to the beginning consonant of the base when the tongue anticipates what sound is coming next. In fact, *ad-* assimilates before lots of consonants, so you may come across it as *ac-*, *af-*, *ag-*, *al-*, *an-*, *ap-*, *ar-*, *as-*, or *at-*, or it may even be shortened just to *a-*. Do not try and memorize the list, just be aware that if you come across a prefix that you do not immediately recognize, it may be an assimilated form.

SUFFIXES

1. -culum	small
2. -tion	act of, process of
3. -ulum	small
4. -ulus	small
5. -uncle	small

BASES

We will look here mostly at the anatomy of the mouth and at things related to the sense of taste. Although speech is delivered through the mouth, we will consider that in the next chapter when we look at the throat and voice box. Remember, we have already seen the base STOM- meaning "mouth, opening," and recall that the base MENT- means "chin" as well as "mind."

1. **OR—mouth, opening**
   OS—mouth, opening

   suboral (*sub*-OR-al) – pertaining to below the mouth

   orad (OR-ad) – toward the mouth

   aborad (*ab*-OR-ad) – toward away from the mouth, i.e., in a direction away from the mouth

   osculum (OS-culum) – small opening, i.e., a pore

2. **GEUS—to taste, sense of taste**

   ageusia (*a*-GEUS-ia) – condition of without sense of taste

   hypergeusesthesia (*hyper*-GEUS-ESTHE-sia) – condition of more than normal sensation to taste

Note that hypergeusesthesia has the format *prefix*-BASE-BASE-suffix. The procedure for building up the term is exactly the same as we used previously for the term hyperphotesthesia. The combination of the base GEUS- with the suffix -ia is a fairly common one; we can add this to our list of compound suffixes.

3. **GUST—to taste**

    gustation (GUST-ation) – process of tasting

    gustatory (GUST-atory) – pertaining to taste

4. **GLOSS—tongue, language**
    GLOTT—(i) tongue, language: (ii) glottis

    glossectomy (GLOSS-ectomy) – surgical removal of the tongue

    glossodynia (GLOSS-odynia) – painful condition of the tongue

    aglossostomia (*a*-GLOSS-O-STOM-ia) – condition of without mouth and tongue

    xenoglossia (XEN-O-GLOSS-ia) – condition of (knowing) a language that is foreign, i.e., the supposed ability to communicate in an unlearned language

    hypoglottal (*hypo*-GLOTT-al) – pertaining to below the tongue, i.e., pertaining to on the underside of the tongue

Like hypergeusesthesia, aglossostomia also has the format *prefix*-BASE-BASE-suffix. The procedure for building up the term is largely the same as we used previously, but common sense dictates some slightly different choices have to be made along the way. Let us go through the process. Start with the suffix, as always; -ia tells us we are dealing with a noun, a "condition." As we did previously, let us forget about the prefix for the moment, since we need to establish the relationship between the bases before we can figure out whether the prefix modifies the penultimate base, the ultimate base, or both. We can be pretty certain that the suffix is applying at least to STOM-, since this is the base closest to it; so, "condition of the mouth (or, opening)." What about the other base, GLOSS-; can the two bases be joined with "and," or is the penultimate base providing extra information such as to "how" or "where" about the ultimate base? Certainly "condition of the mouth and tongue" makes sense, and is more sensible than either "condition of the mouth with the tongue" or "condition of the mouth in the tongue," so let us choose "condition of the mouth and tongue." Now, we have to consider the prefix *a*-, "without"; it must modify both bases, since nothing else makes sense, giving us "condition of without mouth and tongue." We will look at the meaning "glottis" for the base GLOTT- in the next chapter.

5. **LINGU—tongue, language**

    lingual (LINGU-al) – pertaining to the tongue, pertaining to language

    faciolingual (FACI-O-LINGU-al) – pertaining to the tongue and face

    retrolingual (*retro*-LINGU-al) – pertaining to behind the tongue, pertaining to the backward part of the tongue

    sublingual (*sub*-LINGU-al) – pertaining to underneath the tongue

6. PAPILL—nipple, papilla

retinopapillitis (RETIN-O-PAPILL-itis) – inflammation of the (optic) papilla and the retina

papilliferous (PAPILL-I-FER-ous) – pertaining to bearing papillae, i.e., pertaining to having nipples, papules, or pimples

papillectomy (PAPILL-ectomy) – surgical removal of a papilla

Note the combining vowel in papilliferous is "i." Any small, nipplelike projection may be termed a papilla (plural papillae). The tongue is covered with papillae; they give the tongue its characteristic rough texture. There are four types of papillae on the tongue; three of the types house taste buds, the fourth type is concerned with gripping food to help move it around the mouth.

7. FREN—bridle, rein

By extension, the term frenum has the medical meaning of a connecting fold of a membrane that limits the movement between a fixed part and a movable part:

FREN—frenum

frenate (FREN-ate) – having a frenum

frenotomy (FREN-O-tomy) – surgical cutting of a frenum

frenulum (FREN-ulum) – small frenum

In the mouth, there are frenula (plural of frenulum) beneath the tongue, and inside the lower and upper lips.

8. CAR—flesh, meat
CARN—flesh, meat

caruncle (CAR-uncle) – small (piece of) flesh, i.e., a small, fleshy outgrowth

carnose (CARN-ose) – having the quality of flesh

carnophobia (CARN-O-phobia) – abnormal fear of meat

In the mouth, there is a caruncle on either side of the frenulum beneath the tongue.

9. BUCC—cheek

intrabuccal (*intra*-BUCC-al) – pertaining to within the cheek

bucconasal (BUCC-O-NAS-al) – pertaining to the nose and cheeks

buccolingual (BUCC-O-LINGU-al) – pertaining to the tongue and cheeks

10. LABI—lip
LABR—lip

labiate (LABI-ate) – having lips

labioplasty (LABI-O-plasty) – surgical reshaping of the lips

labiograph (LABI-O-graph) – instrument used to measure lip (movement during speaking)

labral (LABR-al) – pertaining to a lip, or liplike part

The term labium can indicate any liplike structure; so, the inner and outer folds either side of the vagina are termed the labia (plural of labium). Likewise, the term labrum may signify a "lip" or "liplike structure."

11. CHEIL—lip

acheilia (*a*-CHEIL-ia) – condition of without a lip or both lips

cheilectomy (CHEIL-ectomy) – surgical removal of a lip

cheilitis (CHEIL-itis) – inflammation of the lip

In case you were wondering, the vertical groove that extends from above the upper lip to the nose is termed the philtrum. The ancient Greeks called it *philtron*, the same word they used for a love charm or potion; remember, we saw the base PHIL- is associated with love. We do not know what prompted the link; perhaps they saw this part of the body as a particularly erogenous zone, or maybe a love potion might be trickled down the philtrum and into the mouth of a sleeping object of desire.

12. STAPHYL—grape, bunch of grapes

We saw previously that the small piece of flesh hanging down at the back of the mouth got the name uvula because of its resemblance to a small grape (UV-ula) on a stem. This was the name given to it by the ancient Romans, but the ancient Greeks also likened the structure to a grape and called it *staphyle*. Today, we rarely see this noun applied to the structure itself—we prefer the term uvula—but the base STAPHYL- occurs fairly often in compound terms related to the uvula:

STAPHYL—uvula

staphylotomy (STAPHYL-O-tomy) – surgical cutting of the uvula

staphyloschisis (STAPHYL-O-SCHI(S)-sis) – condition of a split uvula

Note how the final "s" of the base in staphyloschisis is dropped because the following suffix also begins with an "s."

13. PALAT—roof of the mouth, palate

palatine (PALAT-ine) – pertaining to the palate

palatoglossal (PALAT-O-GLOSS-al) – pertaining to the tongue and palate

palatoschisis (PALAT-O-SCHI(S)-sis) – condition of a split palate, i.e., cleft palate

Note how the final "s" of the base in palatoschisis is dropped because the following suffix also begins with an "s."

14. URAN—roof of the mouth, palate

uranoplasty (URAN-O-plasty) – surgical reshaping of the palate

uranorrhaphy (URAN-O-rrhaphy) – surgical suture of the palate

uranoschisis (URAN-O-SCHI(S)-sis) – condition of split palate, i.e., cleft palate

The medical meaning of this base was in use in ancient Greece; its source is the term *ouranos*, the heavens, but its meaning was extended to include anything that was shaped like the vault of heaven, such as a tent, a ceiling, or the roof of the mouth. Note how the final "s" of the base in uranoschisis is dropped because the following suffix also begins with an "s." The combination of the base SCHI(S)- with the suffix -sis is a very common one; we can add this to our list of compound suffixes.

15. GNATH—jaw

dysgnathic (*dys*-GNATH-ic) – pertaining to abnormal jaw (development)

perignathic (*peri*-GNATH-ic) – pertaining to around the jaw

prognathous (*pro*-GNATH-ous) – having a forward (jutting) jaw, i.e., jaw that projects beyond the upper part of the face

The jaw is the term applied to the bones that contain the teeth, namely the two upper jaw bones and the single lower jaw bone.

16. MAXILL—upper jaw bone, maxilla

admaxillary (*ad*-MAXILL-ary) – pertaining to near the upper jaw bone

hemimaxillectomy (*hemi*-MAXILL-ectomy) – surgical removal of half the upper jaw bone

inframaxillary (*infra*-MAXILL-ary) – pertaining to below the upper jaw bone

17. MANDIBUL—lower jaw bone, mandible

mandibular (MANUDIBUL-ar) – pertaining to the lower jaw bone

mandibulectomy (MANDIBUL-ectomy) – surgical removal of the lower jaw bone

mandibulofacial (MANDIBUL-O-FACI-al) – pertaining to the facial and lower jaw bones

The mandible, or lower jaw, is the only moveable bone in the skull. Processes (bony projections) provide attachment points for muscles and ligaments; each side of the mandible has a coronal process (remember, CORON-al "pertaining to like a crown," i.e., crown shaped) and a condylar process:

18. CONDYL—knuckle, knob

This base refers to the knuckle of a joint, or any hard, bony knob, but you will probably only ever come across it in relation to a condyle, the rounded bump at the end of a bone where it meets with another bone:

CONDYL—condyle

condylar (CONDYL-ar) – pertaining to a condyle

condylectomy (CONDYL-ectomy) – surgical removal of a condyle

condylotomy (CONDYL-O-tomy) – surgical cutting of a condyle

19. RAM—branch

ramiform (RAM-I-form) – having the form of a branch

Note the combining vowel in ramiform is "i." In anatomy, an individual divided part, or branch, of a structure may be termed a ramus. The horizontal part of the mandible extends upward on either side into a mandibular ramus:

RAM—ramus

ramitis (RAM-itis) – inflammation of a ramus

ramulus (RAM-ulus) – small ramus, i.e., terminal branch of a ramus

20. GINGIV—gum

labiogingival (LABI-O-GINGIV-al) – pertaining to the gums and lips

gingivalgia (GINGIV-algia) – painful condition of the gums

gingivoglossitis (GINGIV-O-GLOSS-itis) – inflammation of the tongue and gums

21. DENT—tooth

interdental (*inter*-DENT-al) – pertaining to between the teeth

denticle (DENT-I-cle) – small tooth, i.e., a small tooth or toothlike projection

dedentition (*de*-DENT-I-tion) – process of (becoming) without teeth, i.e., loss of teeth

Note the combining vowel in both denticle and dedentition is "i."

22. ODONT—tooth

endodontics (*end*-ODONT-ics) – study of inside the teeth, i.e., dentistry dealing with teeth roots and dental pulp

odontonecrosis (ODONT-O-NECR-osis) – process of the death of a tooth

23. SALIV—spit, saliva

salivary (SALIV-ary) – pertaining to saliva

salivation (SALIV-ation) – process of (producing) saliva

24. SIAL—spit, saliva, salivary gland

asialia (*a*-SIAL-ia) – condition of without saliva

sialic (SIAL-ic) – pertaining to saliva

sialostenosis (SIAL-O-STEN-osis) – abnormal condition of narrowing of the salivary gland

25. PTY—spit, saliva

ptysis (PTY-sis) – act of spitting

26. PTYAL—saliva, salivary gland

hyperptyalism (*hyper*-PTYAL-ism) – condition of excessive saliva

ptyalogenic (PTYAL-O-genic) – producing saliva

ptyalography (PTYAL-O-graphy) – process of recording salivary gland (form and functioning)

SOME MORE THINGS TO LEARN

We have now seen quite a few suffixes that form the special type of nouns called diminutives, terms that express the small size of the thing in question. You might have noticed that some of these suffixes are very similar, except for their last one or two letters. This is because these different endings indicate whether the noun in question is masculine, feminine, or neuter, something that is very important for both Greek and Latin nouns, hardly important at all for their English translations. Here are some forms we have already come across, and some new ones:

1. -culus, -cula, -culum	small
2. -ellus, -ella, -ellum	small
3. -illus, -illa, -illum	small
4. -ulus, -ula, -ulum	small

These are the remaining suffixes meaning "small" that you are likely to come across in medical terminology; again, some we have already seen, some are new. Memorize them all.

5. -cle	small
6. -idium	small
7. -il	small
8. -ium	small
9. -ole	small
10. -ule	small
11. -uncle	small
12. -unculus	small

Sometimes, the forming of diminutive involves some alteration to the base. For example, the term cerebellum, which actually means "small brain," is a contracted form of the base CEREBR- and the suffix -ellum. Similarly, ocellus, a "small eye" (generally a simple eye, or eyespot), is a contracted form of the base OCUL- and the suffix -ellus.

Since we have now looked at all the diminutive forming suffixes, here are some new bases to learn that indicate size and quantity:

27. MULT—many, much

multicavous (MULT-I-CAV-ous) – full of empty spaces—many (of them), i.e., full of many empty spaces

multidentate (MULT-I-DENT-ate) – having teeth—many of them, i.e., having many teeth

multocular (MULT-OCUL-ar) – pertaining to eyes—many (of them), i.e., having many eyes

Note the combining vowel in both multicavous and multidentate is "i."

28. POLY—many, much

polyblennia (POLY-BLENN-ia) – condition of mucus—much (of it), i.e., condition of excessive mucus

polycoria (POLY-COR-ia) – condition of the pupil of the eye—many (of them), i.e., condition of having more than one pupil in the eye

polyhidria (POLY-HIDR-ia) – condition of sweat—much (of it), i.e., condition of excessive sweating

29. HEMI—half

hemiglossectomy (HEMI-GLOSS-ectomy) – surgical removal of the tongue—half (of it), i.e., surgical removal of one side of the tongue

hemicephalgia (HEMI-CEPH-algia) – painful condition of the head—half (of it), i.e., headache on one side of the head

hemiopalgia (HEMI-OP-algia) – painful condition of the eyes—half (of them), i.e., pain in one eye

Note how we have to apply some common sense here; while pain in half of the head makes sense, pain in half of the eye does not.

30. SEMI—half, partly

semilenticular (SEMI-LENTICUL-ar) – having the character of the lens of the eye (in one) half, i.e., a lens that is convex like the lens of the eye on one side only

The base SEMI- is the Latin equivalent of HEMI- and, in general, is used in compound terms with Latin derived bases, while HEMI- appears in compound terms with Greek-derived bases. The majority of compound terms have Greek origins, so you will not see SEMI- very often in medical terminology.

The first thing you probably noticed about these four bases is that we have already seen the prefixes *multi-*, *poly-*, *hemi-*, and *semi-* with exactly the same meanings. What is going on? Well, if you look up these terms in medical dictionaries, you might find them listed as prefixes, or as bases, or even as both, and these entries might well not agree with entries in regular dictionaries. Sometimes, there is just no agreement as to what constitutes a prefix or a base. From my viewpoint, any word part that indicates size or quantity is almost always derived from an adjective and must, therefore, be classified as a base, and this includes *multi-*, *poly-*, *hemi-*, and *semi-*; remember, prefixes are generally prepositions and adverbs, and bases are adjectives, nouns, or verbs with their endings missing.

So why did I include those four word parts amongst the prefixes? Well, since these four particularly are often cited as prefixes, it gives me an opportunity to bring up this point, and also to illustrate how much like prefixes these parts behave. If we look at the examples above with MULTI-, POLY-, HEMI-, and SEMI-, notice how awkwardly our definitions turn out using our normal procedure for BASE-BASE-suffix terms (suffix first, added to ultimate base, add in penultimate base to make best sense); how much simpler it would be if we thought of them as *prefix*-BASE-suffix type terms and built up the definition accordingly (generally, suffix first, then prefix, and then base). You will find that this is especially true of a lot of terms that include word parts indicating size or quantity. This is due partly to the fact that many of these terms are in regular use in everyday language, as well as in medical and scientific terminology, but also because very often the word part indicating size or quantity comes at the beginning of the term. However, irrespective of this, and irrespective of ease of definition building, you should think of these word parts as bases.

To summarize, then. All the word parts presented here that indicate size and quantity are classified as BASES. Although the initial definition might be awkward, it is still perfectly possible to build up the definition using the regular approach for BASE-BASE-suffix type terms. We will deal with more complicated situations as we come across them.

Here are some new bases that indicate size and quantity:

31. OLIG—few, scanty

olighidrosis (OLIG-HIDR-osis) – abnormal condition of sweating that is scanty

oligoptyalism (OLIG-O-PTYAL-ism) – condition of saliva that is scanty

oligotrichosis (OLIG-O-TRICH-osis) – abnormal condition of the hair that is scanty

32. PLUR—many, more

plurocular (PLUR-OCUL-ar) – pertaining to eyes—many of them

33. PLEO—more, excessive, multiple
PLEIO—more, excessive, multiple

pleochroic (PLEO-CHRO-ic) – pertaining to colors that are multiple

pleocytosis (PLEO-CYT-osis) – abnormal condition of the cells that are excessive (in number), i.e., abnormal condition of more than the normal number of cells

pleiomorphous (PLEIO-MORPH-ous) – pertaining to forms that are many

34. PAN—all, entire
PANT—all, entire

pansclerosis (PAN-SCLER-osis) – abnormal condition of hardening of an entire (organ or part)

panencephalitis (PAN-ENCEPHAL-itis) – inflammation of the brain—all of it, i.e., inflammation of both the gray and white matters of the brain

pantophobia (PANT-O-phobia) – abnormal fear of all things

pantaphobia (PANT-*a*-phobia) – abnormal non-fear of all things, i.e., total fearlessness

Note the almost identical forms of pantophobia and pantaphobia, yet the exact opposite definitions; see how important one letter can be. Pantaphobia is unusual in that a base precedes the prefix. We have already seen the same format in pupillatonia (PUPILL-*a*-TON-ia)—remember, phobia is really PHOB-ia. The method for building up the definition is leave the base that precedes the prefix till last, treat the remaining *prefix*-BASE-suffix in the normal manner (always start with the suffix, then add the prefix, then add in your base) and then add in the other base last. We will see if this works for all terms of this sort as we progress.

35. MACR—large, long

macroblepharia (MACR-O-BLEPHAR-ia) – condition of the eyelid that is (abnormally) large

macrocephalic (MACR-O-CEPHAL-ic) – pertaining to a head that is (abnormally) large

macrognathia (MACR-O-GNATH-ia) – condition of the jaw that is (abnormally) large

36. MAGN—large, great

magnisonant (MAGN-I-SON-ant) – pertaining to a sound that is large

Note the combining vowel in magnisonant is "i."

37. MICR—small

microdontia (MICR-ODONT-ia) – condition of the teeth that are (abnormally) small

microsomia (MICR-O-SOM-ia) – condition of the body that is (abnormally) small

microscopic (MICR-O-SCOP-ic) – pertaining to viewing (something) small

38. MEGA—large, great
MEGAL—large

megaprosopia (MEGA-PROSOP-ia) – condition of the face that is (abnormally) large

megalgia (MEG(A)-algia) – painful condition (that is) great, i.e., a very severe pain

rhinomegaly (RHIN-O-MEGAL-y) – state of an (abnormally) large nose

Both MICR- and MEGA- have very specific meanings in the metric and SI systems of measurement; we will deal with these in a later chapter. Note how the final "a" of the base in megalgia is dropped because the following suffix also begins with an "a." This base and the one that follows are unusual among these size and quantity bases in that they can appear both at the beginning and end of the term. The combination of the base MEGAL- with the suffix -y is a very common one; we can add this to our list of compound suffixes.

39. PEN—deficiency, decrease

penalgesia (PEN-algesia) – sensation of pain decrease, i.e., a reduction in pain points

sarcopenia (SARC-O-PEN-ia) – condition of deficiency of flesh, i.e., loss of muscle mass

lipopenia (LIP-O-PEN-ia) – condition of deficiency of fats (in the body)

leukocytopenia (LEUK-O-CYT-O-PEN-ia) – condition of deficiency of cells that are white, i.e., condition of deficiency of white blood cells

The combination of base PEN- with the suffix -ia is a very common one: we can add this to our list of compound suffixes:

1. -geusia	condition of sense of taste
2. -megaly	enlargement
3. -penia	deficiency
4. -schesis	fissure

In addition, here are some bases that indicate quality:

40. **HOL—whole, entire**

holotrichous (HOL-O-TRICH-ous) – having hair, or hairlike structures, over the entire (body)

holosoamtic (HOL-O-SOMAT-ic) – pertaining to the body—the whole of it, i.e., pertaining to the entire body

41. **HOM—same, similar**
HOME—same, similar

homodontic (HOM-ODONT-ic) – pertaining to teeth that are all the same (in form)

homogenesis (HOM-O-genesis) – production of (offspring) similar (to parents)

homeopathy (HOME-O-pathy) – treatment of disease with similars, i.e., treatment of disease based on the principle that likes are cured by likes

42. **IS—equal, same**

isochromatic (IS-O-CHROM-atic) – pertaining to a color that is the same, i.e., pertaining to a uniform color

isocoria (IS-O-COR-ia) – condition of the pupils being the same (size)

isothymia (IS-O-THYM-ia) – condition of emotion that is equal, i.e., condition of emotional equilibrium

43. **ANIS—unequal, different**

anisocoria (ANIS-O-COR-ia) – condition of the pupils being unequal (in size)

anisognathous (ANIS-O-GNATH-ous) – having jaws of unequal (size)

anisopia (ANIS-OP-ia) – condition of sight that is different (in each eye)

More correctly, ANIS- is a combination of the prefix *an-* ("not") and the base IS-, but it is often treated as a base in its own right.

44. **ALL—other, different**

allesthesia (ALL-ESTHE-sia) – condition of sensation at a different (place from the stimulus)

allochroism (ALL-O-CHRO-ism) – condition of color being different, i.e., condition of change of color of skin or hair

45. **HETER—other, different**

heterodontic (HETER-ODONT-ic) – pertaining to teeth that are different (in form), i.e., pertaining to teeth of varying shape

heterotrichosis (HETER-O-TRICH-osis) – abnormal condition of hair that is different (colors)

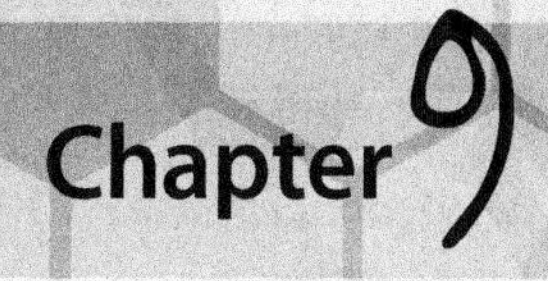

THROAT AND NECK

PREFIXES

There are no more prefixes to learn.

SUFFIXES

1. -acious	tending to, inclined to
2. -ence	state of
3. -ian	pertaining to

BASES

1. CERVIC—neck

cervicalgia (CERVIC-algia) – painful condition of the neck

cervical (CERVIC-al) – pertaining to the neck

In anatomy, the term "neck" is applied to many body parts that have a constricted or narrowed portion. The base CERVIC- may indicate the neck of the uterus, bladder, or tooth, as well as the area between head and torso. You may have to rely on context to figure out which neck is being referred to, or common sense may help you:

cervicobuccal (CERVIC-O-BUCC-al) – pertaining to the cheek (side) of the neck (of a tooth)

Here, for example, the base BUCC- suggests the cheek and mouth area, so there is a pretty good chance that the term is referring to the neck of a tooth. Compare this term:

cervicooccipital (CERVIC-O-OCCIPIT-al) – pertaining to the occiput and the neck

The inclusion of the base for the occiput ("back of the head") guides us toward understanding the neck as the area between head and torso. There are seven cervical bones in the neck area of the spine. The topmost is called the atlas, named after Atlas in Greek mythology, because the bone supports the head just as the god Atlas was made to support the heavens.

2. TRACHEL—neck

trachelodynia (TRACHEL-odynia) – painful condition of the neck

tracheleal (TRACHEL-eal) – pertaining to the neck

Some ambiguity also applies to this base; TRACHEL- may be used about the neck of the uterus (rarely the bladder or tooth), as well as the area between head and torso. Again, common sense can sometimes help:

trachelectomy (TRACHEL-ectomy) – surgical removal of the neck (of the uterus)

It is fairly unlikely that the neck between head and torso would be surgically removed, so here we can safely guess that the neck of the uterus is meant. For this next term, we can apply the same reasoning we used for cervicooccipital:

tracheloocipital (TRACHEL-O-OCCIPIT-al) – pertaining to the occiput and the neck

You may see these terms, cervicooccipital and tracheloocipital, hyphenated as cervico-occipital and trachelo-occipital.

3. COLL—neck

decollate (*de*-COLL-ate) – to (take) away from the neck, i.e., to decapitate, to behead

This base rarely appears in compound terms, but the noun collum is a common anatomical term; like the two previous bases, it can mean the neck between head and torso, or any necklike portion of an organ or structure, especially the narrowed sections of bones. The collarbone, the bone between shoulder and ribcage, takes its common name from this base. You will have to rely on context to help you differentiate this base from the base COLL- meaning "glue."

4. CLEID—key, hook

Because they thought the collarbone was shaped like the hook that fastened a door, the ancient Greeks gave the bone the same name as the hook, *kleis*:

CLEID—collarbone

cleidagra (CLEID-agra) – painful seizure in the collarbone

cleidocranial (CLEID-O-CRANI-al) – pertaining to the cranium and collarbone

cleidotripsy (CLEID-O-TRIPS-y) – act of crushing the collarbone, i.e., act of crushing the collarbones of a fetus to effect delivery

5. CLAV—key, clavicle, collarbone
CLAVICUL—clavicle, collarbone

clavicular (CLAVICUL-ar) – pertaining to the clavicle

subclavian (*sub*-CLAV-ian) – pertaining to below the clavicle

The Romans used the same idea as the Greeks and named the collar-bone *clavicula*, literally "little key." We use the term clavicle today. Both CLAV- and CLAVICUL- are used to denote the clavicle.

6. JUGUL—neck, throat

jugular (JUGUL-ar) – pertaining to the neck or throat

Two pairs of jugular veins return deoxygenated blood from the head and face back to the heart. The two carotid arteries supply the head and face with oxygenated blood. The base CAROT- has nothing to do with the location of the arteries; it comes from the Greek word meaning "to plunge into a deep sleep," since compression of these arteries can cause unconsciousness.

7. GUTTUR—throat

guttural (GUTTUR-al) – pertaining to the throat

gutturonasal (GUTTUR-O-NAS-al) – pertaining to (sound produced from) nose and throat

8. PHARYNG—throat, pharynx

pharyngeal (PHARYNG-eal) – pertaining to the pharynx

pharyngectomy (PHARYNG-ectomy) – surgical removal of the pharynx

pharyngoscope (PHARYNG-O-scope) – instrument used to examine the pharynx

oropharyngeal (OR-O-PHARYNG-eal – pertaining to the oropharynx

The pharynx is the passageway that leads from the nasal and oral cavities toward the larynx (voice box); it is divided into three areas—the nasopharynx, oropharynx, and laryngopharynx.

9. TONSILL—tonsil

tonsillitis (TONSILL-itis) – inflammation of the tonsil

tonsillotome (TONSILL-O-tome) – instrument used to cut the tonsil

peritonsillar (*peri*-TONSILL-ar) – pertaining to around the tonsil

The term tonsil is applied to several structures in the body, but most often refers to the palatine tonsils, the two rounded lumps at the back of the throat. Because of their almondlike shape, these tonsils are sometimes referred to as the amygdalae (remember the base AMYGDAL- meaning "almond").

10. ADEN—gland

polyadenous (POLY-ADEN-ous) – having glands—many of them

adenomegaly (ADEN-O-megaly) – enlargement of a gland

adenoid (ADEN-oid) – resembling a gland

The adenoids are masses of soft tissue at the upper end of the throat behind the nose; they are part of the immune system. They are present at birth and enlarge during childhood, but they tend to shrink during adulthood. Like the palatine tonsils, they are similar to the lymph glands of the neck, armpits, and groin but, as their name suggests, they are not true glands. Their more scientific name is the pharyngeal tonsils.

11. LARYNG—voice box, larynx

laryngeal (LARYNG-eal) – pertaining to the larynx

laryngorrhea (LARYNG-O-rrhea) – (excessive) discharge from the larynx

laryngostenosis (LARYNG-O-STEN-osis) – abnormal condition of narrowing of the larynx

The larynx is that part of the windpipe (airway) where sound production occurs. It is made up from a framework of cartilage and elastic membranes.

12. GLOTT—(i) tongue, language: (ii) glottis, mouth of the windpipe

glottitis (GLOTT-itis) – inflammation of the glottis

infraglottic (*infra*-GLOTT-ic) – pertaining to below the glottis

Located at the upper part of the larynx, the glottis comprises the vocal cords and the space between them. The epiglottis, a lidlike piece of cartilage, folds over the entrance to the windpipe during swallowing so that no food can enter the lungs. Remember, we looked at this base previously, where it had the meaning "tongue."

13. THYR—oblong shield

thyroid (THYR-oid) – resembling an oblong shield

In ancient Greece, the *thyreos* was a shield that was shaped like a door (the term derives from the word for door); Galen used the term thyroid about the cartilage in the larynx that has this oblong form and, in the 17th century, the term was applied to the gland in the neck that is similarly shaped:

THYR—(i) thyroid gland: (ii) thyroid cartilage
THYROID—(i) thyroid gland: (ii) thyroid cartilage

thyromegaly (THYR-O-megaly) – enlargement of the thyroid gland

thyrotomy (THYR-O-tomy) – surgical cutting of the thyroid gland or the thyroid cartilage

thyroiditis (THYROID-itis) – inflammation of the thyroid gland

You will find that most of the compound terms using this base relate to the thyroid gland, simply because it experiences more disorders than does the thyroid cartilage. As always, you will have to rely on common sense and context to help you where there is any ambiguity.

14. HY—Greek letter upsilon (υ)

hyoid (HY-oid) – υ shaped

The υ-shaped bone that supports the tongue got the name hyoid in antiquity because its shape resembles the Greek letter upsilon. The base HY- is used today to indicate this bone:

HY—hyoid bone

hyoglossal (HY-O-GLOSS-al) – pertaining to the tongue and the hyoid bone

hyopharyngeal (HY-O-PHARYNG-eal) – pertaining to the pharynx and the hyoid bone

15. PHAS—speech, to talk

dysphasia (*dys*-PHAS-ia) – condition of abnormal or difficult speech

cryptophasic (CRYPT-O-PHAS-ic) – pertaining to speech that is hidden, i.e., pertaining to speech that is unintelligible to outsiders

16. PHRAS—speech, to talk

polyphrasia (POLY-PHRAS-ia) – condition of speech—much of it, i.e., condition of excessive talkativeness

hypophrasic (*hypo*-PHRAS-ic) – pertaining to less than normal speech, i.e., pertaining to speech that is absent or slower than normal

17. PHEM—speech, to talk

aphemic (*a*-PHEM-ic) – pertaining to without speech

paraphemia (*para*-PHEM-ia) – condition of abnormal speech, i.e., speech using wrong or inappropriate words

18. LAL—speech, to talk

alalia (*a*-LAL-ia) – condition of without speech, i.e., an inability to speak

laliatry (LAL-iatry) – medical treatment of speech (disorders)

lalopathy (LAL-O-pathy) – disease or disorder (affecting) speech

19. LOQU—speech, to talk

multiloquacious (MULTI-LOQU-acious) – tending to speak much

sialoquence (SIA(L)-LOQU-ence) – state of speaking and (producing) saliva, i.e., state of spitting while speaking

Note that the final letter "l" of the base SIAL- has been dropped because the following base also begins with the letter "l." The base LOQU- does not occur very often in medical terminology, although very common in non-technical terms. It does, however, give us a Latin equivalent of a Greek term we mentioned earlier, tragophonia, a condition of the voice that makes it sound like a bleating goat. So, in case you wondered, capriloquism (*capra* is Latin for goat) is the word you want.

20. VOC—speech, voice, to talk

vocal (VOC-al) – pertaining to the voice

Here is another base, again a Latin one, that is more commonly found in non-technical vocabulary. Likewise the base FA-/FANT-, meaning "speech" or "to talk," from which we get the word infant, literally a "non-speaking person."

21. PHON—speech, voice, sound

aphonic (*a*-PHON-ic) – pertaining to without voice

euphonous (*eu*-PHON-ous) – having a good sound

22. LOG—speech, word

dyslogia (*dys*-LOG-ia) – condition of abnormal speech

logorrhea (LOG-O-rrhea) – flow of words, i.e., excessive talkativeness

logamnesia (LOG-*a*-MNE-sia) – condition of without memory of words

adenology (ADEN-O-LOG-y) – act of speech about glands, i.e., the study of glands

Logamnesia is another example of a compound term where a base precedes the prefix. We have already seen pupillatonia and pantaphobia; note that all three involve the prefix *a*-. Exactly the same method for building up the definition can be used here—leave the base that precedes the prefix till last, treat the remaining *prefix*-BASE-suffix in the normal manner (always start with the suffix, then add the prefix, then add in your base) and then add in the other base last. The combination of the base LOG- and the suffix -y is extremely common and we can add -logy to our list of compound suffixes; literally meaning the "act of speech or discourse" about something, it has come to mean "study of." Likewise, LOG- and the suffix -ist gives us the compound suffix -logist, "one who studies."

1. -logist	one who studies
2. -logy	study of

SOME MORE THINGS TO LEARN

Here are some new bases that are regularly associated with bases meaning speech:

23. BRADY—slow

bradylalia (BRADY-LAL-ia) – condition of speech that is (abnormally) slow

bradylogia (BRADY-LOG-ia) – condition of speech that is (abnormally) slow

bradyphasia (BRADY-PHAS-ia) – condition of speech that is (abnormally) slow

bradyphrasia (BRADY-PHRAS-ia) – condition of speech that is (abnormally) slow

24. TACHY—fast

tachylalia (TACHY-LAL-ia) – condition of speech that is (abnormally) fast

tachylogia (TACHY-LOG-ia) – condition of speech that is (abnormally) fast

tachyphasia (TACHY-PHAS-ia) – condition of speech that is (abnormally) fast

tachyphrasia (TACHY-PHRAS-ia) – condition of speech that is (abnormally) fast

25. COPR—dung, filth, feces

coprolalia (COPR-O-LAL-ia) – condition of speech that is filthy, i.e., an uncontrollable use of obscene language

coprophasia (COPR-O-PHAS-ia) – condition of speech that is filthy, i.e., an uncontrollable use of obscene language

coprophemia (COPR-O-PHEM-ia) – condition of speech that is filthy, i.e., an uncontrollable use of obscene language

coprophrasia (COPR-O-PHRAS-ia) – condition of speech that is filthy, i.e., an uncontrollable use of obscene language

26. CAC—bad

cacolalia (CAC-O-LAL-ia) – condition of speech that is bad, i.e., an uncontrollable use of obscene language

27. ECH—returned sound, repetition

echolalia (ECH-O-LAL-ia) – condition of speech repetition, i.e., condition of involuntary repetition of words spoken by others

echophrasia (ECH-O-PHRAS-ia) – condition of speech repetition, i.e., condition of involuntary repetition of words spoken by others

In Greek mythology, the nymph Echo was only able to speak the last words spoken to her by someone else. This was a punishment from Hera, wife of Zeus, because Echo had tried to help Zeus hide his infidelities from his wife. When Echo fell in love with Narcissus, a youth doomed to love only himself, she was unable to tell him her feelings. When Narcissus died, Echo wasted away from sadness, till all that was left of her was her voice, still repeating the last words of others.

In the last chapter, we looked at some bases that indicate size, quantity, and quality. We saw that, in almost all cases, these bases occur at the beginning of a compound term and act almost like prefixes. Here are some bases related to number and quantity; these also occur at the beginning of the term. Remember, you should still deal with the suffix and ultimate base first, and then add in any other bases. The resulting translation may be clumsy, but it will be accurate; you can always make it more elegant once you know exactly what it means.

28. MON—one, single

monesthetic (MON-ESTHE-tic) – pertaining to a sensation—a single one

29. UN—one, single

uniocular (UN-I-OCUL-ar) – pertaining to the eye—one of them

Note the combining vowel in uniocular is "i."

30. HAPL—single

haplopia (HAPL-OP-ia) – condition of sight (that forms a) single (image), i.e., condition of sight where an object viewed by two eyes is seen as a single image

31. PROT—first, original, primitive

protomorphic (PROT-O-MORPH-ic) – pertaining to the shape that is (the most) primitive

32. PRIM—first

primigeneal (PRIM-I-GEN-eal) – pertaining to produced first, i.e., characteristic of the first formation

Note the combining vowel in primigeneal is "i." The terms gravida and para are used about women who have been pregnant or have given birth, respectively. When preceded by a base designating a number, this indicates the number of times a woman has been pregnant (to the stage of viability of the fetus) or has given birth:

primigravida (PRIM-I-gravida) – a woman who has been pregnant for the first time

primipara (PRIM-I-para) – a woman who has given birth for the first time

Note the combining vowel in primigravida and primipara is "i." We will look properly at the bases GRAVID- and PAR- in later chapters. Although they are not true compound suffixes, we will add -para and -gravida to our list.

1. -gravida	woman who is, or has been, pregnant
2. -para	woman who has given birth

33. DI—two, twice
DICH—in two

dicephaly (DI-CEPHAL-y) – condition of the head—two of them (in conjoined twins), i.e., condition of two separate heads in conjoined twins

dichotomy (DICH-O-tomy) – cutting into two, i.e., division into two parts

34. BI—(i) two, twice, double: (ii) life, living
BIN—double, pair

bilabial (BI-LAB-ial) – pertaining to the lips—two of them

binotic (BIN-OT-ic) – pertaining to the ears—a pair of them

We will look at the second meaning of BI- in a later chapter.

35. DEUT—second
DEUTER—second

deutogenic (DEUT-O-GEN-ic) – pertaining to produced second, i.e., pertaining to subsequent formation

deuteropathy (DEUTER-O-pathy) – disease that is second(ary to the initial disease)

36. SECOND—second, following
SECUND—second, following

secondary (SECOND-ary) – pertaining to second (in importance)

secundigravida (SECUND-I-gravida) – a woman who has been pregnant a second time

secundipara (SECUND-I-para) – a woman who has given birth a second time

Note the combining vowel in secundigravida and secundipara is "i."

37. GEMIN—twin, paired, born at the same time
GEMELL—twin, paired, born at the same time

geminate (GEMIN-ate) – having paired (structures)

gemellipara (GEMELL-I-para) – a woman who has given birth to twins

Note the combining vowel in gemellipara is "i."

38. TRI—three

trisulcate (TRI-SULC-ate) – having grooves—three of them

trigeminal (TRI-GEMIN-al) – pertaining to born at the same time—three, i.e., threefold

You will probably only ever come across the term trigeminal in relation to the fifth cranial nerve, which takes the name trigeminal because it is made up of three different branches of nerve.

39. TERTI—third
TERN—three each

tertian (TERTI-an) – pertaining to the third

tertigravida (TERTI-gravida) – a woman who has been pregnant a third time

ternary (TERN-ary) – pertaining to three each, i.e., pertaining to something composed of three units

The term tertian may be used about the third stage of a disease, or to a recurring symptom, which appears every third day inclusively, i.e., every 48 hours. Note the combining vowel in tertigravida is "i." In practice, the more general terms multigravida and multipara are used about women who have been pregnant, or given birth, more than once.

40. TETR—four

tetramastous (TETR-A-MAST-ous) – having breasts—four (of them)

Note the combining vowel in tetramastous is "a."

41. QUADR—four

quadritubercular (QUADR-I-TUBERCUL-ar) – pertaining to tubercles—four (of them)

Note the combining vowel in quadritubercular is "i." This term is generally used about molar teeth that have four tubercles or cusps

42. QUART—fourth
QUATERN—four each

quartan (QUART-an) – pertaining to the fourth

quartigravida (QUART-I-gravida) – a woman who has been pregnant a fourth time

quaternary (QUATERN-ary) – pertaining to four each, i.e., pertaining to something composed of four units

Quartan is another term used about a recurring symptom; this time, one which appears every four days inclusively, i.e., every 72 hours. Note the combining vowel in quartigravida is "i."

43. PENT—five

pentapterous (PENT-A-PTER-ous) – having wings—five (of them)

Not a term you are really likely to encounter in human medical terminology, but it gets the idea across. We have not met the base DACTYL- ("finger, toe") yet, but you will find pentadactyly (PENT-A-DACTYL-y) is a term in medical terminology—"condition of the fingers or toes—five (on each hand or foot)." If we think of the meaning "digit" for the base DAC-TYL-, we can get around the problem of four fingers and a thumb. Note the combining vowel in pentapterous is "a."

44. QUINQUE—five

quinquetubercular (QUINQUE-TUBERCUL-ar)—pertaining to tubercles—five (of them)

Again, a term used about molar teeth.

45. QUINT—fifth
QUIN—five each

quintan (QUINT-an) – pertaining to the fifth, i.e., recurring every five days inclusively

quintipara (QUINT-I-para) – a woman who has given birth a fifth time

quinary (QUIN-ary) – pertaining to five each, i.e., pertaining to something composed of five units

Note the combining vowel in quintipara is "i."

You are unlikely to come across the bases for the numbers beyond five in medical terminology, but I include them here, just for completeness. Where I could find no medical term that uses them, I have used a suffix common in mathematics, -gon (from the base GON- meaning "angle, corner" familiar in the term polygon, for a geometrical figure with many angles.

46. HEX—six

hexagon (HEX-A-gon) – (geometrical figure with) six angles

Note the combining vowel in hexagon is "a."

47. SEX—six

sexdigitate (SEX-DIGIT-ate) – having digits—six (of them)

We have not met the base DIGIT- yet, meaning "fingers, toes," but it seem to be one of the few medical terms that uses the base SEX-.

48. SEXT—sixth

sextan (SEXT-an) – pertaining to the sixth, i.e., recurring every six days inclusively

sextigravida (SEXT-I-gravida) – a woman who has been pregnant a sixth time

Note the combining vowel in sextigravida is "i."

49. HEPT—seven

heptachromic (HEPT-A-CHROM-ic) – pertaining to colors—seven (of them)

Used about the ability to see the seven colors of the spectrum. Note the combining vowel in heptachromic is "a."

50. SEPT—(i) dividing wall: (ii) seven

septan (SEPT-an) – pertaining to seven, i.e., recurring every six days inclusively

septigravida (SEPT-I-gravida) – a woman who has been pregnant seven times

Note the combining vowel in septigravida is "i." Note also the subtle change; the term uses the base for the cardinal number SEPT- (seven) as opposed to the base for the ordinal number (seventh). There is some inconsistency with the formation of the terms using -para and -gravida with the larger numbers. Be careful not to confuse this base with SEPT- meaning "dividing wall" that we saw in a previous chapter; you will have to rely on context to help you.

51. SEPTIM—seventh

septimal (SEPTIM-al) – pertaining to the seventh (in a series)

52. OCT—eight

octan (OCT-an) – pertaining to eight, i.e., recurring every eight days inclusively

octipara (OCT-I-para) – a woman who has given birth eight times

Note the combining vowel in octipara is "i."

53. OCTAV—eighth

I can find no compound terms using this base, but the eighth cranial nerve is sometimes called the octavus nerve.

54. ENNE—nine

enneagon (ENNE-A-gon) – (geometrical figure with) nine angles

More commonly called a nonagon. Note the combining vowel in enneagon is "a."

55. NOVEM—nine

November.

All I could come up with. The original Roman calendar had ten months, and *November* was the ninth month (preceded by *QUINTilis*, *SEXTilis*, *SEPTember*, and *OCTober* and followed by *DECember*).

56. NON—ninth

nonipara (NON-I-para) – a woman who has given birth a ninth time

Note the combining vowel in decipara is "i."

57. DEC—ten

decagon (DEC-A-gon) – (geometrical figure with) ten angles

Note the combining vowel in decagon is "a."

58. DECEM—ten

December

59. DEC—tenth
DECIM—tenth

decigravida (DEC-I-gravida) – a woman who has been pregnant a tenth time

Note the combining vowel in decigravida is "i." In Roman times, if a group of soldiers were guilty of some crime such as treason or mutiny, their commanders might choose to decimate the group as punishment— killing one tenth of the number.

One last thing. Here are the most common bases used in the metric and SI systems of measurement. You do not need to memorize them, but it is good to be aware of them. Remember, the bases MICR- and MEGA- also have the meanings "small" and "large," respectively.

MEGA-	million 10^6
KILO-	thousand 10^3
HECT-	hundred 10^2
DECA-	ten 10^1
DECI-	tenth 10^{-1}
CENTI-	hundredth 10^{-2}
MILLI-	thousandth10^{-3}
MICR-	millionth 10^{-6}

The bases CENTI- and MILLI- are unusual in that they have other meanings, "hundred" and "thousand," in everyday language. A century, for example, is one hundred years, a millennium one thousand years, while a centipede traditionally (though not actually) has one hundred legs, a millipede one thousand legs.

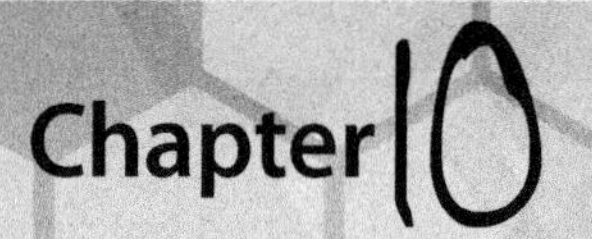

SHOULDERS AND ARMS

SUFFIXES

1. -ated	composed of, having

BASES

1. **SCAPUL—shoulder blade, scapula**

    scapular (SCAPUL-ar) – pertaining to the shoulder blade

    scapulodynia (SCAPUL-ODYN-ia) – condition of pain in the shoulder blade

The medical term for the shoulder blade, the large triangular bone that lies at the back of the ribs, is the scapula (plural scapulae).

2. **BRACHI—arm**

    brachiocephalic (BRACHI-O-CEPHAL-ic) – pertaining to the head and arm

    cervicobrachial (CERVIC-O-BRACHI-al) – pertaining to the arm and neck

    macrobrachia (MACR-O-BRACH(I)-ia) – condition of the arm that is (abnormally) large

Notice how the final "i" of BRACHI- in macrobrachia has been dropped because the following suffix also begins with "i."

3. **MEL—limb**

amelia (*a*-MEL-ia) – condition of without a limb

erythromelalgia (ERYTHR-O-MEL-algia) – painful condition of a limb (accompanied by) redness of the part

megalomelia (MEGAL-O-MEL-ia) – condition of a limb that is (abnormally) large

The word limb generally refers to arms and legs, although sometimes the term may be expanded to include other jointed appendages (hands, fingers, feet, and toes).

4. **HUMER—upper arm bone, humerus**

humeral (HUMER-al) – pertaining to the upper bone of the arm

The medical term for the upper arm bone is the humerus.

5. **ULN—ulna**

ulnad (ULN-ad) – toward the ulna

ulnar (ULN-ar) – pertaining to the ulna

The ulna is the longer of the two bones of the lower arm (connected at the little finger side at the wrist)

6. **RADI—ray, spoke of a wheel, radius**

radiate (RADI-ate) – to (extend like) spokes of a wheel, i.e., to spread out in all directions from the center

radiodermatitis (RADI-O-DERMAT-itis) – inflammation of the skin (caused by exposure to) rays (of electromagnetic radiation)

radioulnar (RADI-O-ULN-ar) – pertaining to the ulna and radius

As well as its other meanings, this base means "radius" both in the sense of a line extending from the center of a circle to its periphery, and the shorter of the two bones of the lower arm (connected at the thumb side at the wrist). All four of the terms, scapula, humerus, ulna, and radius were used by ancient Romans, though not necessarily with the exact precision that we use them today. Both the humerus and the ulna got their names from Greek equivalents. The radius bone may have got its name because it rotates around the ulna at both the elbow and wrist, or because it has some resemblance to an ancient weaving shuttle, which was another meaning of the term radius. The term for the pointy bit of the elbow is the olecranon, which gets its name from the Greek forms of ulna and cranium, because it is actually the head (or skull) of the ulna bone.

7. **CUB—to lie down**
   CUBIT—to lie down
   CUMB—to lie down

   cubation (CUB-ation) – process of lying down

   decubital (*de*-CUBIT-al) – pertaining to (occurring) from lying down

   procumbent (*pro*-CUMB-ent) – pertaining to forward lying down, i.e., lying face down

A decubitus ulcer, or bedsore, occurs because of lying down too long in the same position. Since ancient Romans ate their meals lying down but propped up on one elbow, the elbow, and sometimes the forearm, got the name cubitum:

CUBIT—elbow, forearm

cubital (CUBIT-al) – pertaining to the elbow or forearm

brachiocubital (BRACHI-O-CUBIT-al) – pertaining to the elbow and arm

8. **ANCON—elbow**

   anconad (ANCON-ad) – toward the elbow

   anconitis (ANCON-itis) – inflammation of the elbow

   anconeal (ANCON-eal) – pertaining to the elbow

Anconeal (or anconal) may also mean pertaining to the anconeus muscle, a muscle that stabilizes the elbow during rotation.

9. **GLEN—socket of a joint**

   glenoid (GLEN-oid) – resembling a socket of a joint

Probably the only time you will come across the base GLEN- is in relation to the shoulder. The shallow depression on the scapula that engages with the head of the humerus bone is termed the glenoid (sometimes the glenoid fossa or glenoid cavity):

GLEN—glenoid

glenohumeral (GLEN-O-HUMER-al) – pertaining to the humerus and the glenoid

10. **CORAC—crow's beak**

    coracoid (CORAC-oid) – resembling a crow's beak

Likewise, probably the only time you will come across the base CORAC- is in relation to the shoulder. The coracoid process on the scapula gets its name because it has the shape of a crow's beak (remember, a process is a bony projection that provides attachment points for muscles and ligaments):

CORAC—coracoid process

coracoclavicular (CORAC-O-CLAVICUL-ar) – pertaining to the clavicle and the coracoid process

11. ACROMI—acromion

subacromial (*sub*-ACROMI-al) – pertaining to below the acromion

acromioclavicular (ACROMI-O-CLAVICUL-ar) – pertaining to the clavicle and the acromion

The spine of the scapula (a bony projection) runs obliquely across the posterior surface; the acromion, or acromial process, lies at its lateral end, where it forms a joint with the clavicle and provides an attachment point for ligaments and muscles. The term was already in use with the ancient Greeks and means, literally, "extremity of the shoulder."

12. CAPIT—head
CIPIT—head

capitate (CAPIT-ate) – having a head(shape)

capitulum (CAPIT-ulum) – small head

capitellum (CAPIT-ellum) – small head

In an earlier chapter, we came across the base OCCIPIT- with the meaning the "back of the head" or, more technically, the "occiput." The term derives from this base, CIPIT-, and the prefix *ob*-, meaning literally "against the head." Notice how *ob*- has assimilated to *oc*- in front of the letter "c" in CIPIT-. Most medical compound terms involving the head use the base CEPHAL-, while you will find CAPIT- and CIPIT- more often in everyday English language (think of capital, decapitate, and precipitate for example). Capitulum and capitellum, "the small heads" generally refer to headlike structures, such as the head or extremity of a bone. In Latin, the terms biceps and triceps mean "two-headed" and "three-headed," respectively, with the form CEPS being closely related to the base CAPIT- "head." Since the two major muscles of the upper arm have two and three "heads" (the head of a muscle is its fixed point or origin, as opposed to the moveable point of insertion), the terms were adopted to describe them, the biceps being on the anterior side of the upper arm, the triceps on the posterior. More correctly, the muscles are the biceps brachii and the triceps brachii, the "biceps of the arm" and "triceps of the arm," since there are other two- and three-headed muscles in the body; the leg, in fact, not only has biceps and triceps muscles, but also has a quadriceps.

bicipital (BI-CIPIT-al) – pertaining to heads—two of them, pertaining to the biceps

tricipital (TRI-CIPIT-al) – pertaining to heads—three of them, pertaining to the triceps

Ancient medical writings were often presented in *a capite ad calcem* manner, literally "from head to heel." The writers would start by discussing topics related to the head and then proceed down the body. We would call it, "from head to toe"; this book is presented in *a capite ad calcem* manner.

13. DELT—Greek letter delta (Δ)

deltoid (DELT-oid) – shaped like the Greek letter delta

The deltoid is the large triangular muscle at the rounded part of the shoulder, extending to the upper arm. In anatomy, the term delta may be used about a flat triangular surface.

14. TRAPEZ—table

trapezoid (TRAPEZ-oid) – resembling a table

trapezium (TRAPEZ-ium) – small table

The ancient geometrists developed the term *trapezium* for a four-sided figure with no parallel sides from the Greek word for a small table. In anatomy, a trapezium (or sometimes trapezius) is a structure with that shape:

TRAPEZI—trapezium

trapeziform (TRAPEZI-form) – having the form of a trapezium

trapeziectomy (TRAPEZI-ectomy) – surgical removal of the trapezium

The trapezius muscle is a roughly diamond-shaped muscle extending from the neck, across the shoulders, and down the spine. The trapezium bone is an irregularly shaped bone of the hand; trapeziectomy is performed on this bone, not on the muscle.

Here are some other bases that refer to, or are used about, muscles, bones, and tissues in general, including those of the arms and shoulders.

15. OST—bone
OSTE—bone

dysostosis (*dys*-OST-osis) – condition of abnormal bone (formation)

osteopenia (OSTE-O-penia) – deficiency of bone (density)

osteolipochondroma (OSTE-O-LIP-O-CHONDR-oma) – tumor of the cartilage (made up of) fat and bone tissue

The term osteolipochondroma has three bases, but approach it in the same way that we have approached terms with two bases. Begin with the suffix and the ultimate base—that gets the definition off to the proper start and we know whether we are dealing with a noun, adjective, or verb. Then, we have to consider the other two bases. Can we just use the word "and" to link them with the ultimate base? It is possible, but unlikely that tumors of all three tissues would occur at the same time and, if they did, we would probably be looking at a specific condition in which that combination of tumors occurred. So, as always, we have to think of the most likely common sense solution.

16. TEND—to stretch
TENS—to stretch
TENT—to stretch

extendable (*ex*-TEND-able) – able to be out stretched, i.e., able to be stretched out

tensor (TENS-or) – thing that stretches

extensor (*ex*-TENS-or) – thing that out stretches, i.e., thing that stretches out

distention (*dis*-TENT-ion) – condition of apart stretching, i.e., being stretched apart

A muscle that stretches some part of the body is a tensor muscle. A muscle that extends or straightens a body part is an extensor muscle; the triceps is an extensor muscle in the arm. We also get the word "tendon" from this base, the name for the tough fibrous bands of tissue that connect muscles to bones. The base for the term tendon has a challenging number of alternative forms:

17. TEN—tendon
TEND—tendon
TENDIN—tendon
TENDON—tendon
TENON—tendon
TENONT—tendon

tenodynia (TEN-odynia) – painful condition of a tendon

tendotomy (TEND-O-tomy) – surgical cutting of a tendon

tendinoplasty (TENDIN-O-plasty) – surgical reshaping of a tendon

tendonitis (TENDON-itis) – inflammation of a tendon

tenonectomy (TENON-ectomy) – surgical removal of a tendon

tenontology (TENONT-O-logy) – study of tendons

18. LIG—to bind, to tie

ligature (LIG-ature) – system composed of (something) to bind, i.e., something tied around a structure to constrict it

ligate (LIG-ate) – to bind (something), i.e., to apply a ligature

ligation (LIG-ation) – process of applying a ligature

The bands of fibrous connective tissue that bind bones to other bones are called ligaments. We can think of LIGAMENT- as a base:

19. LIGAMENT—ligament

ligamentary (LIGAMENT-ary) – pertaining to ligament

osseoligamentous (OSSE-O-LIGAMENT-ous) – pertaining to ligament and bone

20. DESM—band, ligament

desmitis (DESM-itis) – inflammation of a ligament

desmopathy (DESM-O-pathy) – disease of the ligaments

While the term ligament (or the Latin *ligamentum*) is generally used about the structure itself, the Greek base DESM- is more commonly found denoting a ligament in compound terms. It is related to the base DE- we saw previously, meaning "to bind." You will often find the combination of the prefix *syn-* with the base DESM-; literally meaning a "banding together," SYNDESM- is often used as a base meaning ligament:

21. SYNDESM—ligament

syndesmorrhaphy (SYNDESM-O-rrhaphy) – surgical suture of a ligament

syndesmotomy (SYNDESM-O-tomy) – surgical cutting of a ligament

22. FASCI—band, fascia

fasciation (FASCI-ation) – process of (applying) bands, i.e., process of binding with bandages

fasciectomy (FASCI-ectomy) – surgical removal of (strips of) a fascia

fasciodesis (FASCI-O-desis) – surgical fusion of a fascia (to a tendon or other fascia)

A fascia is a band or sheet of fibrous connective tissue enclosing, or separating, muscles and organs.

23. MY—muscle
MYS—muscle
MYOS—muscle

myalgia (MY-algia) – painful condition of a muscle

myogenesis (MY-O-genesis) – production of muscle (cells or tissue)

myopathy (MY-O-pathy) – disease of muscle (tissue)

epimysial (*epi*-MYS-ial) – pertaining to on the surface of a muscle, i.e., pertaining to the fibrous covering of a muscle

myositis (MYOS-itis) – inflammation of a muscle

The ancient Greek word for muscle, from which we get this base, is also the word for a mouse. Supposedly, there is some resemblance between the shape of certain muscles and mice, so that is why the muscle got its name.

24. MUSCUL—muscle

intramuscular (*intra*-MUSCUL-ar) - pertaining to within the muscle

cervicomuscular (CERVIC-O-MUSCUL-ar) - pertaining to the muscles of the neck

musculature (MUSCUL-ature) - system composed of muscles

The Romans followed Greek usage in this case, and the Latin for muscle uses the same word as that for "little mouse"; you will come across this term, *musculus*, in anatomy.

25. FLECT—to bend
FLEX—to bend

reflection (*re*-FLECT-ion) - act of bending backward, i.e., in anatomy, act of bending or folding back of a part upon itself

flexion (FLEX-ion) - act of bending

flexor (FLEX-or) - thing that bends

A muscle that bends a body part is a flexor muscle; the biceps is a flexor muscle in the arm.

26. AGON—struggle, contest, action

agonism (AGON-ism) - condition of action

antagonism (*ant*-AGON-ism) - condition of opposite action, i.e., condition of an opposition between forces

agony (AGON-y) - state of struggle, i.e., state of intense pain

Note how the final "i" of *anti-* in antagonism has been elided before the vowel of the base. When a muscle causes a movement to occur, it is called an agonist muscle; when a muscle opposes movement, either slowing movement down or returning body parts to their original position, it is called an antagonist muscle. A muscle can change roles depending on the movement involved. Often, agonist and antagonist muscles work together in what are called antagonistic pairs, where one muscle contracts as the other relaxes; the biceps and triceps of the arm are an antagonistic pair of muscles.

27. DUC—to lead, to draw
DUCT—to lead, to draw

abducent (*ab*-DUC-ent) – pertaining to away from (the midline) drawing, i.e., pertaining to drawing away

adduction (*ad*-DUCT-ion) – act of toward (the midline) drawing, i.e., act of a movement of a body part toward the midline of the body

circumduction (*circum*-DUCT-ion) – act of around drawing, i.e., act of the circular movement of a body part

A muscle that draws a body part away from the midline of the body is called an abductor; one that draws a body part toward the midline is called an adductor.

28. LAMIN—thin plate, lamina

laminar (LAMIN-ar) – pertaining to a lamina (thin plate), or having the character of laminae (thin plates)

laminated (LAMIN-ated) – composed of laminae (thin plates)

laminitis (LAMIN-itis) – inflammation of a lamina (thin plate)

There are numerous structures throughout the body that are called laminae because of their thin, platelike appearance. The term lamella is a diminutive form:

29. LAMELL— thin plate, lamella

lamellar (LAMELL-ar) – pertaining to a lamella (thin plate), or having the character of lamellae (thin plates)

Bone lamellae form the basic structural unit of bone.

30. ARTHR—(i) joint: (ii) speech

arthritis (ARTHR-itis) – inflammation of a joint

arthropathology (ARTHR-O-PATH-O-logy) – study of the diseases of joints

dysarthria (*dys*-ARTHR-ia) – condition of abnormal speech, i.e., condition of difficult or unclear speech

The two meanings of this base were already related in ancient Greek, since both joints and speech were viewed as made up of distinct parts (bones or words) coming together to make the whole. As always, you will have to rely on context to help you decide which meaning is required.

31. ARTICUL—(i) joint: (ii) speech sound

interarticular (*inter*-ARTICUL-ar) – pertaining to between joints

articulation (ARTICUL-ation) – process of being jointed, process of (forming) speech sounds

disarticulation (*dis*-ARTICUL-ation) – process of separate joint, i.e., process of separation at a joint, amputation

biarticulate (BI-ARTICUL-ate) – having joints–two (of them)

The two meanings of this base also occurred in the Latin language.

32. CRIST—crest

cristate (CRIST-ate) – having a crest

intercristal (*inter*-CRIST-al) – pertaining to between crests

In anatomy, a crest, or crista (plural cristae), is an elevated ridge. A ridge or elevation on a bone may be termed a crest.

33. PHY—to grow
PHYS—(i) growth, nature: (ii) breath, inflation, swollen

physis (PHY-sis) – process of growing

physics (PHYS-ics) – science of nature

physocephaly (PHYS-O-CEPHAL-y) – state of head (being) swollen

epiphysis (*epi*-PHY-sis) – condition of upon (the rest) growing, i.e., condition of an area of secondary formation

diaphysis (*dia*-PHY-sis) – condition of in a line growing, i.e., condition of an area of formation from one end to another

It is not easy to see at first what these last two terms mean. They refer to the structure of long bones of the arms and legs; the diaphysis is the long shaft of bone extending from one end to the other, capped top and bottom by an epiphysis, an area of bone that is initially separate from the shaft and only fuses with it at a later stage. The degree of epiphyseal (*epi*-PHYS-eal—"pertaining to an epiphysis") fusion between the epiphysis and the diaphysis in skeletal remains can be used as an indication of age, since total fusion does not generally occur before late teens or early twenties. Once you know that these terms are related to bone structure, figuring out that a symphysis (*sym*-PHY-sis) is a fusing together of bone, and that an apophysis (*apo*-PHY-sis) is an outgrowth of bone becomes easier. Again, you will have to rely on context to help you decide which meaning is required for the base PHYS-.

34. SPIN—thorn, spine

spinate (SPIN-ate) – having spines

spinalgia (SPIN-algia) – painful condition of the spine

infraspinous (*infra*-SPIN-ous) – pertaining to below a spine

The link was already made in the ancient world between thorns and spines on plants to spines on animals and fish, and, ultimately, to any spinelike structure in humans. Today, spine is not only the everyday word for the vertebral column or backbone, but any slender, straight projection or ridge may be termed a spine in anatomy. The spine of the scapula is a bony process that extends obliquely across its posterior surface.

SOME MORE THINGS TO LEARN

Here are some more bases to learn; they all have common compound suffixes associated with them that indicate some sort of medical condition:

35. TOP—place, position

topophobia (TOP-O-phobia) – abnormal fear of (certain) places

dystopic (*dys*-TOP-ic) – pertaining to abnormal position (of a body part)

ectopia (*ec*-TOP-ia) – condition of outside the (correct) position, i.e., condition of displacement

adenectopy (ADEN-*ec*-TOP-y) – condition of outside the (correct) position gland, i.e., condition of displacement of a gland

In adenectopy, we have another term where a base precedes the prefix. We have already seen logamnesia, pupillatonia, and pantaphobia; all three involved the prefix *a*-. Now we have a term with the prefix *ec*-, but exactly the same method for building up the definition can be used here—leave the base that precedes the prefix till last, treat the remaining *prefix*-BASE-suffix in the normal manner (always start with the suffix, then add the prefix, and then add in your base) and then add in the other base last.

36. TA—to stretch
TAS—stretching, tension

iridotasis (IRID-O-TA-sis) – condition of stretching the iris (of the eye)

entasia (*en*-TAS-ia) – condition of inward tension, i.e., a spasm

ectasia (*ec*-TAS-ia) – condition of outward stretching, i.e., widening or expansion

37. EDE—to swell
OEDE—to swell

edesis (EDE-sis) – condition of swelling

The base EDE- (OEDE- is just an alternative spelling) is unusual in that you will probably never come across it other than in the combination EDEma (OEDEma), which is actually an unmodified Greek noun meaning "swelling," and not a true BASE-suffix combination. It is probably better to think of it only as one of the compound suffixes:

arthredema (ARTHR-edema) – swelling of the joints

lipedema (LIP-edema) – swelling (caused by subcutaneous) fat

The tragic Greek hero Oedipus supposedly got his name (the Greek form literally means "swollen-footed") from his scarred and swollen feet, the result of his parents having had his feet bound and pierced as an infant to prevent him returning home after being abandoned.

38. EME—to vomit

antiemetic (*anti*-EME-tic) – pertaining to against the act of vomiting, i.e., pertaining to preventing vomiting

hyperemesis (*hyper*-EME-sis) – condition of more than normal vomiting, i.e., condition of excessive vomiting

dysemesia (*dys*-EME-sia) – condition of painful vomiting

39. PHRAG—to block, to obstruct

emphraxis (*em*-PHRAG-sis) – condition of inward blocking, i.e., condition of obstruction

laryngemphraxis (LARYNG-*em*-PHRAG-sis) – condition of inward blocking of the larynx, i.e., condition of obstruction or closure of the larynx

adenemphraxis (ADEN-*em*-PHRAG-sis) – condition of inward blocking of a gland, i.e., condition of obstruction in a gland

In adenemphraxis, we have another term where a base precedes the prefix. Use exactly the same method for building up the definition as we did previously—leave the base that precedes the prefix till last, treat the remaining *prefix*-BASE-suffix in the normal manner (always start with the suffix, then add the prefix, and then add in your base) and then add in the other base last. Remember that *en*- becomes *em*- before the letter "p" because of the process of assimilation; note also that the final "g" of the base and the "s" of the suffix have been combined into the letter "x" to make the "gs" sound easier. The ancient Greek term *diaphragma* meaning a "wall, partition," was also applied to the muscle that divides the chest from the abdomen. In modern terminology, the term diaphragm is used about a variety of thin partitions. We can think of DIAPHRAGM- as a base:

40. DIAPHRAGM—diaphragm

diaphragmatic (DIAPHRAGM-atic) – pertaining to a diaphragm

diaphragmalgia (DIAPHRAGM-algia) – painful condition of the diaphragm

41. LEP—taking hold, to seize
LEPS—taking hold, to seize

analeptic (*ana*-LEP-tic) – pertaining to an upward taking hold, i.e., pertaining to a restorative remedy that strengthens or stimulates

psycholepsy (PSYCH-O-LEPS-y) – state of seizure of the mind, i.e., state of sudden depression

catalepsy (*cata*-LEPS-y) – state of complete seizure, i.e., state of seizure with total loss of voluntary movement

42. MALAC—soft

malacodermous (MALAC-O-DERM-ous) – pertaining to skin that is soft

malacosarcosis (MALAC-O-SARC-osis) – condition of (muscular) tissue that is (abnormally) soft

osteomalacia (OSTE-O-MALAC-ia) – condition of softening of the bones

craniomalacia (CRANI-O-MALAC-ia) – condition of softening of the cranium

43. PHTHI—to waste away, to decay
PHTHIS—wasting, decay

ophthalmophthisis (OPHTHALM-O-PHTHI-sis) – condition of decay of the eye

laryngophthisis (LARYNG-O-PHTHI-sis) – condition of wasting in the larynx

phthisic (PHTHIS-ic) – pertaining to wasting

44. PLEG—blow, stroke

glossoplegia (GLOSS-O-PLEG-ia) – condition of stroke of the tongue, i.e., condition of paralysis of the tongue

quadriplegic (QUADR-I-PLEG-ic) – pertaining to a stroke of the four (limbs), i.e., pertaining to paralysis of all four limbs

prosopodiplegia (PROSOP-O-DI-PLEG-ia) – condition of stroke on two sides of the face, i.e., condition of paralysis of both sides of the face

Note the combining vowel in quadriplegic is "i." Closely related to this base is:

PLEX—blow, stroke, seizure

PLEC—blow, stroke, seizure

cataplexy (*cata*-PLEX-y) – condition of down stroke, i.e., condition of falling-down seizure

phrenoplexia (PHREN-O-PLEX-ia) – condition of seizure of the mind, i.e., condition of a trancelike state

cataplectic (*cata*-PLECT-ic) – pertaining to down stroke, i.e., pertaining to a falling-down seizure

The term phrenoplexia is outdated now, but you may still come across it. Remember, the base PHREN- has two meanings, "mind" and "diaphragm"; we have to use context and common sense to decide which is the most appropriate. The term apoplexia was already used by the ancient Greeks for a form of madness or seizure. It is now a fairly obsolete medical description for a cerebral stroke, but the term still persists in everyday language, usually in the form apoplexy, to denote a fit of extreme anger. You must be careful not to confuse this base with the base PLEX- we will meet later on, which means "to interweave" or "to fold together."

45. PTO—falling

proptosis (*pro*-PTO-sis) – condition of forward falling, i.e., condition of forward protrusion, usually of the eye

blepharoptosis (BLEPHAR-O-PTO-sis) – condition of falling of the eyelid, i.e., condition of drooping eyelid

glossoptosia (GLOSS-O-PTO-sia) – condition of falling of the tongue, i.e., condition of drooping of the tongue

46. STA—to stand, standing
STAS—standing

astasia (*a*-STA-sia) – condition of not standing, i.e., condition of inability to stand

coprostasis (COPR-O-STA-sis) – condition of standing of the feces, i.e., condition of stoppage of feces evacuation

stasiphobia (STAS-I-phobia) – abnormal fear of standing (and walking)

isostasy (IS-O-STAS-y) – condition of standing equal, i.e., condition of equilibrium

Note the combining vowel in stasiphobia is "i."

47. STHEN—strength

hypersthenia (*hyper*-STHEN-ia) – condition of more than normal strength

asthenia (*a*-STHEN-ia) – condition of without strength, i.e., condition of weakness

anisosthenic (*anis*-O-STHEN-ic) – pertaining to unequal strength (in paired muscles)

Here are the compound suffixes that occur using these bases. Note that asthenia is actually a prefix, base, and suffix combination. Remember, it is helpful to memorize all the compound suffixes because they occur so regularly, but you can also always build them up from their individual base and suffix parts. We can also add -stenosis to this list, which we have seen a few times now in previous chapters.

1. -asthenia	weakness
2. -ectasia, -ectasis	expansion, widening, dilation
3. -ectopia, -ectopy	displacement
4. -emesia, -emesis	vomiting
5. -emphraxis	obstruction
6. -lepsis, -lepsy	seizure
7. -malacia	softening
8. -(o)edema	swelling
9. -phthisis	wasting
10. -plegia	paralysis
11. -plexia, -plexy	seizure
12. -ptosia, -ptosis	drooping, prolapse
13. -stasia, -stasis, -stasy	stoppage, stagnation
14. -stenosis	narrowing, contraction

We have covered another five chapters since the last review, so this seems like a good place for another summary of some of the topics we have covered.

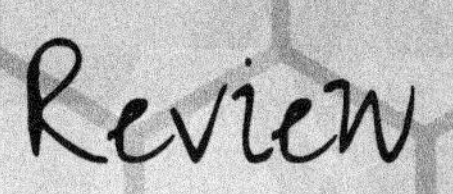

CHAPTERS 6–10

PREFIXES

We have now covered all of the prefixes that you are likely to come across. Most of them are prepositions that indicate where something occurs; a few others indicate how something is done, or have the meaning of "not." Note that *hemi-*, *multi-*, *poly-*, and *semi-* are no longer listed as prefixes (check Chapter 8 if you cannot remember why).

1. *a-, an-*	without, not, non-
2. *ab-, a-*	away from
3. *ad-, ac-, af-* etc.	toward, near
4. *ambi-, ambo-*	both
5. *amphi-, ampho-*	both, on both sides
6. *ana-, an-*	up, upward, again
7. *ante-*	before, in front of
8. *anti-, ant-*	against, opposite
9. *apo-, ap-*	away from
10. *cata-, cat-*	down, complete
11. *circum-*	around
12. *con-, col-, com-, cor-*	together, with
13. *contra-*	opposite, against
14. *de-*	down, downward, away from, from, without, out of

15. *dia-, di-*	through, apart, in a line
16. *dis-, dif-, di-*	apart, away from, separation, lack of
17. *dys-*	bad, painful, difficult, abnormal
18. *ec-, ex-*	out, outside
19. *ecto-, ect-*	outside, outer
20. *eiso-, eso-*	inward
21. *en-, el-, em-, er-*	in, inward
22. *enanti-*	opposite
23. *endo-, end-*	inside, inner
24. *ento-, ent-*	inside, within
25. *epi-, ep-*	upon, on the surface
26. *eu-*	good, well, normal
27. *ex-, ef-, e-*	out, outside, from, without
28. *exo-, ex-*	outside, outer, external
29. *extra-, extro-*	outside of, beyond
30. *hyper-*	over, above, more than normal
31. *hypo-, hyp-*	below, deficient, less than normal
32. *in-, il-, im-, ir-*	in, into
33. *infra-*	below
34. *inter-*	between
35. *intra-*	within
36. *juxta-*	close to
37. *mal-*	bad, inadequate
38. *meso-*	middle
39. *meta-, met-*	after, change, transition

40. *non-*	not
41. *ob-*	toward, in front of, against
42. *para-, par-*	beside, beyond, abnormal
43. *per-*	through
44. *peri-*	around, near
45. *pre-, prae-*	in front of, before
46. *post-*	behind, after
47. *pro-*	in front of, forward
48. *pros-*	toward
49. *re-*	again and again, backward
50. *retro-*	behind, backward
51. *se-*	away, aside
52. *sub-, suc-, sug-, sup-, sur-*	below, underneath
53. *super-*	upper, above, beyond
54. *supra-*	above
55. *syn-, syl-, sym-, sys-, sy-*	together, with, concurrent
56. *trans-*	across, through
57. *ultra-*	beyond

We have seen three ways in which the spelling of the prefix might be altered, depending on the first letter of the base that follows it:

i. Elision—occurs with certain prefixes that end in a vowel. When the following base begins with a vowel or the letter "h," the final vowel of the prefix is dropped. Since the prefix *a-* is nothing other than a vowel, it adds a letter and becomes *an-*. Not all prefixes that end in a vowel undergo elision, and the process is not always consistent even with those prefixes that can undergo elision.

ii. Assimilation—occurs with certain prefixes that end in a consonant. When the following base begins with certain consonants, the final consonant of the prefix changes to something closer to the beginning consonant of the base.

iii. The prefixes *ec-* and *ex-*. The prefix *ec-* also has the alternative form *ex-* that is used before vowels and the letter "h." The prefix *ex-* also undergoes some changes; as a general rule, *ex-* before vowels, the letter "h," and some consonants, *ef-* before "f," and *e-* before most consonants. Luckily, these two prefixes have pretty much the same meaning.

Do be aware of the potential spelling changes. Then, if you come across a prefix that you do not immediately recognize, think whether it could be an elided or assimilated form. Remember, too, that some prefixes just have alternative forms.

SUFFIXES

There are many, many, many suffixes that you might come across, but maybe you will only ever come across them once. Here, we are learning the suffixes that get used over and over. We have already met a lot of them, but we will still continue to add to the list for a few more chapters.

ADJECTIVE-FORMING SUFFIXES

All of these suffixes form an adjective when added to a base:

1. -able, -abil-	able to be
2. -ac	pertaining to
3. -aceous	pertaining to, belonging to, having
4. -acious	tending to, inclined to
5. -ad	toward
6. -al, -eal, -ial	pertaining to
7. -alis, -aris	pertaining to
8. -an	pertaining to
9. -ant	pertaining to
10. -ar	pertaining to, having the character of
11. -ary	pertaining to

12. -ate	pertaining to, having, having the shape, to (...)
13. -ated	composed of, having
14. -atic	pertaining to
15. -atory	pertaining to
16. -ent	pertaining to
17. -escent	beginning to be, becoming
18. -etic	pertaining to
19. -fic	causing, making
20. -form	having the form of, like
21. -ian	pertaining to
22. -iatic	pertaining to a state, pertaining to a process
23. -ible, -ibil-	able to be
24. -ic	pertaining to
25. -ical	pertaining to
26. -id	pertaining to, having
27. -ile	pertaining to, able to be
28. -ine	pertaining to
29. -ior	pertaining to
30. -ive	pertaining to, tending to
31. -oid	resembling, shaped, like, shaped like
32. -ory	having the function of
33. -ose	full of, having the quality of
34. -ous	pertaining to, like, full of, having
35. -tic	pertaining to
36. -ual	pertaining to

Remember, the suffix -ate can also be a verb-forming suffix meaning "to do, to cause."

NOUN-FORMING SUFFIXES

All of these suffixes form a noun when added to a base:

37. -ance, -ancy	state of
38. -ation	process
39. -ature	system composed of
40. -duct	duct, channel, tube
41. -ema	condition
42. -ence	state of
43. -er	person who (does...), thing that (does...)
44. -esis	condition, abnormal condition, process
45. -ety	condition, state, quality
46. -gen	that which produces
47. -gram	record
48. -graph	instrument used to record
49. -ia	condition of, quality of, state of, act of
50. -iasis	state of, process of, abnormal condition
51. -ician	specialist
52. -ics, -tics	art of, science of, study of
53. -in	substance
54. -ion	action, condition, act of
55. -ism	condition of
56. -ist	person who (does...), specialist
57. -itis	inflammation
58. -ity	condition, state, quality
59. -ization	process of making
60. -ment	action of, product of

61. -meter	instrument used to measure
62. -oma	tumor, mass
63. -or	person who (does…), thing that (does…)
64. -orium	place for
65. -osis	process of, condition of, abnormal condition of
66. -plasm	formed substance, growth
67. -scope	instrument used to examine
68. -sia, -sis	process of, condition of, act of
69 -um	structure, substance
70. -ure	result of, act of
71. -y	condition of, quality of, state of, act of

These diminutive-forming suffixes also make nouns when added to a base:

72. -cle	small
73. -culus, -cula, -culum	small
74. -ellus, -ella, -ellum	small
75. -idium	small
76. -il	small
77. -illus, -illa, -illum	small
78. -ium	small
79. -ole	small
80. -ule	small
81. -ulus, -ula, -ulum	small
82. -uncle	small
83. -unculus	small

VERB-FORMING SUFFIXES

All of these suffixes form a verb when added to a base:

84 -ate	pertaining to, having, having the shape, to (...)
85. -esce	to begin, to become
86. -ize	to make, to affect
87. -verse	to turn, to travel turned

Remember, the suffix -ate can also be an adjective-forming suffix.

COMPOUND SUFFIXES

Some base-suffix pairs occur together so regularly that they are often treated as one suffix, and we have used the term compound suffix to describe them. Here are the compound suffixes that we have seen, but bear in mind that this is just a list created for this present task in medical terminology. In a different discipline, the list of compound suffixes would be quite different.

Remember, it is helpful to memorize all the compound suffixes because they occur so regularly, but you can also always build them up from their individual base and suffix parts.

Most of the compound suffixes we have made are nouns. Here are the ones that relate to the senses and the mind:

1. -acousia	condition of hearing
2. -blepsia	condition of sight
3. -esthesia	condition of sensation
4. -geusia	condition of sense of taste
5. -mania	condition of madness, compulsion, obsession
6. -mnesia	condition of memory, memory
7. -opia	condition of sight
8. -opsia	condition of sight

9. -osmia	condition of sense of smell
10. -philia	condition of attraction, abnormal craving for
11. -phobia	condition of fear, abnormal fear of

Here are the ones that relate to medical procedures and treatment:

12. -centesis	surgical puncturing, puncturing
13. -clasia, -clasis	surgical fracture, breaking, rupture
14. -cleisis	surgical closure, closure
15. -clysis	therapeutic infusion of liquid, irrigation
16. -desis	surgical fusion, binding
17. -dialysis	surgical dissolving, surgical separation, filtration
18. -ectomy	surgical removal, removal
19. -iatrics, -iatry	medical treatment
20. -lysis	surgical dissolving, surgical separation, loosening
21. -pexis, -pexy	surgical fastening, fixing
22. -plasia, -plasty	surgical reshaping, formation
23. -stomy	making a surgical opening, making an opening
24. -therapia, -therapy	treatment
25. -tripsy	surgical crushing, crushing
26. -tomy	surgical cutting, cutting

Here are the ones that express some physical condition:

27. -agra	pain, painful seizure
28. -algesia	sensation of pain
29. -algia	painful condition
30. -asthenia	weakness

31. -ectasia, -ectasis	expansion, widening, dilation
32. -ectopia, -ectopy	displacement
33. -emesia, -emesis	vomiting
34. -emphraxis	obstruction
35. -lepsis, -lepsy	seizure
36. -malacia	softening
37. -megaly	enlargement
38. -nosia	disease
39. -odynia	painful condition
40. -(o)edema	swelling
41. -pathia, -pathy	disease, treatment of disease
42. -penia	deficiency
43. -phthisis	wasting
44. -plegia	paralysis
45. -plexia, -plexy	seizure
46. -ptosia, -ptosis	drooping, prolapse
47. -schisis	fissure
48. -stasia, -stasis, -stasy	stoppage, stagnation
49. -stenosis	narrowing, contraction

The -rrh compounds are not true compound suffixes in the way we have described them, but they do occur quite often, so it is good to be aware of them:

50. -rrhage	excessive flow, excessive discharge
51. -rrhagia	excessive flow, excessive discharge
52. -rrhaphy	surgical suture
53. -rrhea	flow, discharge
54. -rrhexis	rupture

Here are the remaining compound suffixes that form nouns:

55. -cyte	cell
56. -genesis	production
57. -graphy	process of recording
58. -gravida	woman who is, or has been, pregnant
59. -logist	one who studies
60. -logy	study of
61. -metry	process of measuring
62. -para	woman who has given birth
63. -scopy	process of examining with an instrument
64. -tome	instrument used to cut

These compound suffixes form adjectives:

65. -genic	producing, produced
66. -genous	producing, produced
67. -verse	to turn, to travel, turned

BUILDING UP MEDICAL DEFINITIONS

This is a good time to review what we have learned so far about building up medical definitions.

COMBINING VOWELS

Remember, combining vowels do not add anything to the sense of the term. We have seen that "o" is the most common of the combining vowels, but that other vowels can perform this function too. You may have noticed that certain bases and suffixes are always preceded by a particular combining vowel; FER-, -form, and -fic, for example, are always preceded by the letter "i" as a combining vowel. From now on, we will not remark on the combining vowels.

BASE-suffix (INCLUDING ANY TERMS WITH COMBINING VOWELS)

Start with the suffix—this is going to tell you whether your compound term is a noun, adjective, or verb. Then, add the base, and add any little words such as "the" or "of" that you need to make sense.

BASE-BASE-suffix, BASE-BASE-BASE-suffix ETC. (INCLUDING ANY TERMS WITH COMBINING VOWELS)

Many compound terms have more than one base, and they can be the hardest terms to deal with because the relationship between the bases is not always clear. Sometimes, you can join the bases with the word "and," sometimes not. You really have to think about the most likely common sense solution. Practice will help you a lot, as you will start to see certain patterns emerging with particular combinations of suffixes and bases.

Always start with the suffix and the ultimate (last) base—this gets the definition off to the proper start and we know whether we are dealing with a noun, adjective, or verb. Then, use common sense to figure out how to add in the other base(s). In general, and this is not a hard-and-fast rule but I do try to use it if I can, address the bases in turn reading from right to left (end to start, if you prefer). Add in any little words such as "the" or "of" that you need to make sense.

If any of the other bases in a compound term, other than the ultimate base, are adjectival in nature, i.e. describing words that denote quality, size, and quantity, you may end up with a fairly clumsy definition, something like "having digits—six (of them)." This is fine; you can always adjust the word order later to make it sound better, if necessary. However, do adhere to the method outlined for your initial building up of the definition. It is very tempting to treat these adjectival bases as prefixes, but this can cause problems in more complicated compound terms.

BASE-suffix-suffix, BASE-BASE-suffix-suffix ETC. (INCLUDING ANY TERMS WITH COMBINING VOWELS)

Occasionally, there are two suffixes at the end of a term. Make a single suffix from the two, starting with the ultimate (last) one; this will still tell you whether your compound term is a noun, adjective, or verb. Then proceed as normal.

BASE-suffix-BASE-suffix (INCLUDING ANY TERMS WITH COMBINING VOWELS)

Very occasionally a term may have two suffixes, one at the end of the term and the other somewhere in the middle. The only term we have come across like this is acousticophobia, but, because it includes what we have classified as a compound suffix, we looked at it as a BASE-suffix-suffix type term, ACOUS-tic-O-phobia. If we think of -phobia in its original BASE and suffix form, we have ACOUS-tic-O-PHOB-ia. The best approach here is to think of the term as two BASE-suffix units, linked by a hyphen. Start with the last BASE-suffix unit, using the regular method; again, this gets the definition off to the proper start and we know whether we are dealing with a noun, adjective, or verb. Then, work on the other BASE-suffix unit with the regular method. Finally, join the two halves together, adding in any little words such as "the" or "of" that you need to make sense.

prefix-BASE-suffix (INCLUDING ANY TERMS WITH COMBINING VOWELS)

Start with the suffix, then add the prefix, and then add in your base. Add in any words necessary to make good sense. Remember, the prefix adds extra information about the base.

prefix-BASE-BASE-suffix (INCLUDING ANY TERMS WITH COMBINING VOWELS)

These compound terms can be awkward, because it is not always obvious which of the bases the prefix is modifying. The best approach is usually to leave the prefix till last, and build up the definition in the manner outlined for BASE-BASE-suffix type terms. Always start with the suffix and the ultimate (last) base, and use common sense to figure out how to add in the other base. Then, you really have to think about the prefix. We have already seen examples where it modifies both bases, as in aglossostomia, and where it modifies just one, as in hyperphotesthesia and hypergeusesthesia (the ultimate base in both cases). Again, you have to use common sense to decide what works best. Finally, add in any little words such as "the" or "of" you need to make sense. We will talk about other terms of this type as we meet them.

prefix-prefix-BASE-suffix (INCLUDING ANY TERMS WITH COMBINING VOWELS)

In most cases, always start with the suffix, then add the first prefix, then the second prefix, and then add in your base. Add in any words necessary to make good sense.

RULE-BREAKERS AND ODDITIES

We have now seen four examples of terms where a base precedes the prefix; pupillatonia, pantaphobia, logamnesia, and adenectopy. We used the same method in each case—leave the base that precedes the prefix till last, treat the remaining *prefix*-BASE-suffix in the normal manner (always start with the suffix, then add the prefix, and then add in your base) and then add in the other base last.

We will continue to talk about other rule-breakers and oddities as we meet them.

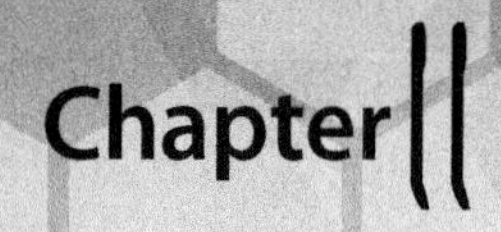

HANDS AND FINGERS

SUFFIXES

1. -ator	person who (does…), thing that (does…)
2. -ious	pertaining to

BASES

1. **CHEIR—hand**
   CHIR—hand

   acheiria (*a*-CHEIR-ia) – condition of (being) without hands

   cheiralgia (CHEIR-algia) – painful condition of the hand

   chiromegaly (CHIR-O-megaly) – enlargement of the hand or hands

2. **MAN—(i) frenzy: (ii) hand: (iii) thin, loose**

   bimanous (BI-MAN-ous) – having hands—two (of them)

   sinistromanual (SINISTR-O-MAN-ual) – pertaining to the hand—the left one, i.e., being left-handed

We have already seen this base with the meaning "frenzy"; we will look at the meanings "thin, loose" in a later chapter.

3. **PALM—palm of the hand**

   palmar (PALM-ar) – pertaining to the palm of the hand

   palmaris (PALM-aris) – pertaining to the palm of the hand

4. **CARP—wrist**

   carpoptosis (CARP-O-ptosis) – drooping of the wrist (due to paralysis)

   metacarpal (*meta*-CARP-al) – pertaining to after the wrist, i.e., pertaining to between the wrist and the fingers

There are eight carpal bones in each wrist, arranged in two rows of four. Five metacarpal bones extend from the wrist, one to the base of each of the fingers and the thumb.

Here is a strange compound term:

carpocarpal (CARP-O-CARP-al) – pertaining to the area between two bones of the wrist

You would probably never figure out the definition of this term without knowing that compound terms that duplicate the same base denote two parts of that structure and the associated area between them. Just something you have to remember.

5. **DACTYL—finger, toe**

   polydactyly (POLY-DACTYL-y) – condition of the fingers or toes—many of them, i.e., condition of more than the normal number of fingers or toes

   dactyledema (DACTYL-edema) – swelling of the fingers or toes

   hyperdactylia (*hyper*-DACTYL-ia) – condition of more than normal (number of) fingers or toes

The combinations of the base DACTYL- with the suffix -y and with the suffix -ia are very common; we will add these to our list of compound suffixes.

6. **DIGIT—finger, toe, digit**

   digital (DIGIT-al) – pertaining to a finger or toe

   sexdigitism (SEX-DIGIT-ism) – condition of the digits—(having) six (per hand or foot)

   digitiform (DIGIT-I-form) – having the form of a finger or toe

Note that the term digitalis can be a bit misleading. In medical terminology, it generally refers to the digitalis plant (so-called because of its fingerlike flowers), or to the active compound contained in its leaves. Digitalism is the term used for the symptoms that accompany poisoning by digitalis.

7. PHALANG—phalanx, finger bone, toe bone

phalangeal (PHALANG-eal) – pertaining to a finger or toe bone, or to a phalanx

symphalangia (*sym*-PHALANG-ia) – condition of together finger or toe bones, i.e., condition of end-to-end fusion of any of the finger or toe bones

tetraphalangeate (TETR-A-PHALANG-E-ate) – having finger or toe bones—four (of them)

The thumb and the big toe each have two bones, the other fingers and toes have three bones each; so, being tetraphalangeate means you have extra finger or toe bones. The anatomical term for each bone is a phalanx (plural phalanges). The bones got this name because they line up in the hand and foot like the lines of Greek soldiers in battle order, the original Greek *phalanx*. Other anatomical structures that involve parts being lined up are also sometimes termed a phalanx.

8. POLLIC—thumb, pollex

pollical (POLLIC-al) – pertaining to the thumb

pollicization (POLLIC-ization) – process of making (a substitute) thumb

The anatomical term for the thumb is the pollex (plural pollices).

9. ACR—highest point, extreme, extremity

acrophobia (ACR-O-phobia) – abnormal fear of high places

acromania (ACR-O-mania) – condition of madness that is extreme, i.e., condition of incurable insanity

acrocyanosis (ACR-O-CYAN-osis) – abnormal condition of blue discoloration of the extremities

acroleukopathy (ACR-O-LEUK-O-pathy) – disease (involving) white (patches on) the extremities

acrocephalopolysyndactyly (ACR-O-CEPHAL-O-POLY-*syn*-DACTYL-y) – condition of together fingers or toes—many of them, and a head that is (like) the highest point, i.e., condition involving several fused fingers or toes and a head that is peak shaped

It will probably take you a few moments to figure out this last term. Not only do we have four bases, but we have a prefix that is nowhere near the beginning of the term. However, as always, start with the suffix. Then, since the prefix is preceding the ultimate base, it is almost certain that the prefix is adding information about this base only, and we can treat this *prefix*-BASE-suffix triplet as if it is a compound term in isolation. In fact, just as we noted above that DACTYL- and -y and -ia are common combinations, so too are *syn*-DACTYL-y and *syn*-DACTYL-ia, literally a "condition of together fingers or toes," more sensibly "a fusion of fingers or toes." Now we have to address the other three bases. Often going from right to left with the bases works; it does here—it is much more likely that we are talking about "many fingers or toes," than "many extremities" or "many heads." So, "a condition of many fused fingers or toes." Can we join in the other two bases with "and"? Not really, this would not make a lot of sense. How about joining in one base with "and"? That works, especially if we still work from right to left; "a condition of many fused fingers or toes and a head ..." Then, if we cannot include ACR- with "and," all we can do is use common sense. Given its position in the term, it is more likely related to CEPHAL- than to DACTYL-, so we can probably think that it is modifying "head" in some way. With a little leap of faith, we arrive at "head that is (like) the highest point," i.e., "cone shaped" or "peak shaped." Again, not easy, but not impossible.

The "extremities" may include any of, or all of, the hands, fingers, feet, and toes.

10. PRON—face downward, bending forward

pronate (PRON-ate) – to turn (to a) face downward (position)

pronation (PRON-ation) – the process of bending forward

pronator (PRON-ator) – thing that bends forward

A pronator muscle turns a body part to the prone (lying face downward, bent forward) position. Pronation of the palm of the hand moves it from a front facing position to a rear facing position (or, to a downward facing position, if the elbow is flexed).

11. SUPIN—face upward, bending backward

supinate (SUPIN-ate) – to turn (to a) face upward (position)

supination (SUPIN-ation) – process of bending backward

supinator (SUPIN-ator) – thing that bends backward

A supinator muscle turns a body part to the supine (lying face upward, bent backward) position. Supination of the palm of the hand moves it from a rear facing position to a front facing position (or, to an upward facing position, if the elbow is flexed).

12. THIGM—to touch, touching
THIX—touching

thigmesthesia (THIGM-esthesia) – condition of sensation to touch

thixotropy (THIX-O-TROP-y) – condition of turning (in response to) touching

13. HAPH—touching
HAPT—to touch, touching

haphalgesia (HAPH-algesia) – painful condition (caused by) touching

haptometer (HAPT-O-meter) – instrument used to measure (sensitivity to) touch

14. TACT—(i) to touch, touching: (ii) order, arrangement
TAG—to touch, touching
TANG—to touch, touching

tactile (TACT-ile) – pertaining to (the sense of) touch

contagious (*con*-TAG-ious) – pertaining to together touching, i.e., pertaining to disease transmission through touching together

tangible (TANG-ible) – able to be touched, i.e., real, not imaginary

The original concept of "contagion" precedes modern notions of a communicable disease. We will look at the meaning "order, arrangement" for the base TACT- in a later chapter.

SOME MORE THINGS TO LEARN

Here are some new bases to learn. They are mostly derived from adjectives so, like the bases that indicate size, quantity, and quality, these bases often occur at the beginning of a compound term. They seem to be like prefixes, but remember, they are bases. You should still deal with the suffix and ultimate base first, then add in any other bases. The resulting translation may be clumsy, but it will be accurate; you can always make it more elegant once you know exactly what it means.

15. DOLICH—long

dolichostenomelia (DOLICH-O-STEN-O-MEL-ia) – condition of the limbs that are narrow and long, i.e., condition marked by abnormally long and slender hands, fingers, feet, and toes

dolichomorphic (DOLICH-O-MORPH-ic) – pertaining to a shape that is (abnormally) long, i.e., pertaining to a body type that is especially long and slender

dolichonychia (DOLICH-ONYCH-ia) – condition of the nails that are (abnormally) long

16. LONG—long

longilingual (LONG-I-LINGU-al) – pertaining to the tongue—a long one

The Latin base LONG- is used more often in botany and non-human zoology; the Greek base DOLICH- is generally used to denote "long" in terminology relating to humans.

17. BRACHY—short

brachydactylia (BRACHY-dactylia) – condition of the fingers that are (abnormally) short

brachyglossal (BRACHY-GLOSS-al) – pertaining to a tongue that is (abnormally) short

brachycheilia (BRACHY-CHEIL-ia) – condition of lips that are (abnormally) short

18. BREV—short

brevilingual (BREV-I-LINGU-al) – pertaining to the tongue—a short one

Like the base LONG-, the Latin base BREV- is used more often in botany and non-human zoology; the Greek base BRACHY- is generally used to denote "short" in terminology relating to humans.

19. EURY—wide

eurygnathism (EURY-GNATH-ism) – condition of the jaw (being) wide

eurycephalic (EURY-CEPHAL-ic) – pertaining to the head that is wide

20. PLATY—flat, broad

platycephalic (PLATY-CEPHAL-ic) – pertaining to a head that is flat

platyglossal (PLATY-GLOSS-al) – pertaining to a tongue that is broad

platyrrhiny (PLATY-RRHIN-y) – condition of the nose (being) broad

Remember, the base -RRHIN- occurs only in the middle of terms; elsewhere the base meaning nose is RHIN-.

21. PACHY—thick

acropachydermic (ACR-O-PACHY-DERM-ic) – pertaining to skin that is thickened at the extremities

pachyblepharosis (PACHY-BLEPHAR-osis) – abnormal condition of the eyelid (being) thickened

pachyotia (PACHY-OT-ia) – condition of the ear (being) thickened

22. PYCN—thick, dense
PYKN—thick, dense

pyknophrasia (PYKN-O-PHRAS-ia) – condition of speech (characterized by) thickness or clumsiness

pyknodysostosis (PYKN-O-*dys*-OST-osis) – condition of abnormal bone (structure characterized by) thickening

The alternative spelling PYCN- (where the "k" of the Greek form is replaced by "c") is occasionally used. In pyknodysostosis, we have another compound term where a prefix is within the word. See the discussion above on the term acrocephalopolysyndactyly.

23. GRAV—heavy

gravimetric (GRAV-I-METR-ic) – pertaining to measurement by heaviness

The term gravid, meaning literally "heavy (with child)" or more commonly "pregnant," is related to this base:

24. GRAVID—pregnant, pregnancy

gravidic (GRAVID-ic) – pertaining to pregnancy or a pregnant woman

gravidity (GRAVID-ity) – condition of pregnancy

We have used the term gravida in a previous chapter, meaning a "pregnant woman."

25. BAR—weight, pressure
BARY—heavy

baresthesia (BAR-esthesia) – condition of sensation to weight or pressure

baranesthesia (BAR-*an*-esthesia) – condition of non-sensation to weight or pressure

bariatrics (BAR-iatrics) – medical treatment of weight, i.e., medical management of obesity

baryphony (BARY-PHON-y) – condition of speech that is heavy, i.e., condition of a heavy, deep voice, or speech that is heavy and indistinct

In baranesthesia, we have another example of an oddity, a BASE-*prefix*-BASE-suffix type compound term (remember, -esthesia is a compound suffix made from a base and suffix). We can use exactly the same method we have seen previously for this type of term—leave the base that precedes the prefix till last, treat the remaining *prefix*-BASE-suffix in the normal manner (always start with the suffix, then add the prefix, and then add in your base) and then add in the other base last.

26. LEPT—thin, slender

leptocephaly (LEPT-O-CEPHAL-y) – condition of the head (being) narrow

leptodactylous (LEPT-O-DACTYL-ous) – pertaining to fingers or toes that are slender

leptorrhinism (LEPT-O-RRHIN-ism) – condition of the nose (being) slender

Remember, the base -RRHIN- occurs only in the middle of terms; elsewhere the base meaning nose is RHIN-.

27. LEI—smooth

leiodermia (LEI-O-DERM-ia) – condition of the skin (being abnormally) smooth

leiomyoma (LEI-O-MY-oma) – tumor (derived from the) muscle that is smooth

leiomyosarcoma (LEI-O-MY-O-SARC-oma) – tumor of the soft tissue (derived from) muscle that is smooth

Muscle tissue is classified into three types; smooth, cardiac, and skeletal. Smooth muscle is generally involuntary, meaning it is not under our conscious control, and is found in places such as blood vessels, the stomach, and the intestines. Remember, a sarcoma (SARC-oma) is a malignant (cancerous) tumor; many tumors are benign (non-cancerous).

28. MOLL—soft

mollescent (MOLL-escent) – becoming soft

mollipilose (MOLL-I-PIL-ose) – having the quality of hair that is soft

You may also come across the term mollities, which means "characterized by softness."

29. DUR—hard

induration (*in*-DUR-ation) – process of in (a place) hardening, i.e., condition of hardening, usually of organs or tissues

We have already met the Greek base SCLER- meaning "hard"; you are much more likely to come across it in compound terms than the Latin base DUR-. However, we do find DUR- in the term dura mater; literally "hard mother," it is a tough membrane that surrounds the brain and spinal cord, the outermost of the three meningeal layers:

DUR—dura mater

dural (DUR-al) – pertaining to the dura mater

duraplasty (DUR-A-plasty) – surgical reshaping of the dura mater

duroarachnitis (DUR-O-ARACHN-itis) – inflammation of the arachnoid and the dura mater

Remember, we came across the arachnoid in a previous chapter; it is the meningeal layer that resembles a spiderweb and it lies beneath the dura mater. The innermost of the three meningeal layers is the pia mater (literally, "tender mother").

30. ORTH—straight, correct

orthodontics (ORTH-ODONT-ics) – science of teeth correction or straightening, i.e., branch of dentistry correcting abnormal tooth position

orthomelic (ORTH-O-MEL-ic) – pertaining to limb correction or straightening

anorthographic (*an*-ORTH-O-GRAPH-ic) – pertaining to writing (that is) not straight or correct, i.e., pertaining to the loss of the ability to write correctly

It is fairly straightforward in anorthographic to figure out which base the prefix *an-* is modifying.

31. ANKYL—bent, stiff, fixed

ankylodactyly (ANKYL-O-dactyly) – condition of the fingers or toes (being) fixed together, i.e., fusion of the fingers or toes

ankylosis (ANKYL-osis) – abnormal condition of stiffening (of a joint)

ankylostomatic (ANKYL-O-STOMAT-ic) – pertaining to the mouth (being) fixed, i.e., pertaining to lockjaw, a closing of the jaw and mouth due to spasm

The alternative spelling ANCYL- (where the "k" of the Greek form is replaced by "c") is only occasionally used.

32. KYPH—bent, humpbacked

kyphosis (KYPH-osis) – abnormal condition of (being) humpbacked

kyphorrhinotic (KYPH-O-RRHIN-O-tic) – pertaining to a nose that is bent

The alternative spelling CYPH- (where the "k" of the Greek form is replaced by "c") is only occasionally used.

33. LORD—bent backward

lordosis (LORD-osis) – abnormal condition of (being) bent backward, i.e., condition of abnormal curvature of the spine

lordotic (LORD-O-tic) – pertaining to (being) bent backward

34. SCOLI—curved, bent

scoliosis (SCOLI-osis) – abnormal condition of (being) curved, i.e., condition of abnormal curvature of the spine

scoliokyphosis (SCOLI-O-KYPH-osis) – abnormal condition of (being) humpbacked and curved, i.e., condition of being humpbacked as well as having an abnormal curvature of the spine lordoscoliosis (LORD-O-SCOLI-osis) – abnormal condition of (being) curved and bent backward, i.e., condition of abnormal curvature of the spine

The alternative spelling SKOLI- is occasionally used.

35. CYRT—curved, bent
KYRT—curved, bent

kyrtometer (KYRT-O-meter) – instrument used to measure curved (surfaces of the body)

cyrtosis (CYRT-osis) – abnormal condition of (being) curved, i.e., condition of abnormal curvature of the spine

You will find both spellings, KYRT- and CYRT-, for this base. Both scoliosis and cyrtosis are characterized by a lateral curvature of the spine. This sideways curve may be "C" or "S" shaped. Kyphosis is characterized by an abnormally rounded upper back, while lordosis is characterized by a significant inward curve of the spine in the lower back area.

36. CAMP—to bend, bent
CAMPT—to bend, bent
CAMPYL—bent, curved

acampsia (*a*-CAMP-sia) – condition of not bending, i.e., condition of stiffness or rigidity of a joint

camptomelia (CAMPT-O-MEL-ia) – condition of the limbs (being) bent, i.e., condition of deformity characterized by curvature of the long bones

camptodactyly (CAMPT-O-dactyly) – condition of the fingers or toes (being) bent

campylognathia (CAMPYL-O-GNATH-ia) – condition of the jaw (being) curved, i.e., a curved deformity of the jaw

Finally, here are the compound suffixes to add to our list:

1. -dactylia, -dactyly	condition of the fingers or toes
2. -syndactylia, -syndactyly-	condition of fused fingers or toes

Chapter 12

CHEST, BACK, AND SPINE

SUFFIXES

1. -fication	process of producing, process of becoming, process of making
2. -fy	to produce, to become, to make

BASES

1. **RACHI—spine, backbone**
   RACHID—spine, backbone
   -RRHACH—spine, backbone

   rachioplegia (RACHI-O-plegia) – paralysis of the spine
   rachischisis (RACHI-schisis) – fission of the spine
   rachidial (RACHID-ial) – pertaining to the spine

The base RHACHI-, which is closer to the Greek original, has largely been replaced by the form RACHI-, but you may still come across it occasionally. You might also come across the form -RRHACH-, which only occurs in the middle of a term, never at the beginning, as in hematorrhacis, the term for a spinal hemorrhage (you have not met the base HEMAT- yet). We looked at the explanation for this unusual form in an earlier chapter, when we looked at the bases RHAPH- and RHE-.

2. **VERTEBR—spine, vertebra**

    vertebral (VERTEBR-al) – pertaining to a vertebra, or vertebrae

    vertebrectomy (VERTEBR-ectomy) – surgical removal of a vertebra

    craniovertebral (CRANI-O-VERTEBR-al) – pertaining to the vertebrae and the cranium

The spinal column is made up of thirty-three vertebrae (singular vertebra), the bones that are linked together to form the backbone, or spine. The term vertebra is related to the base VERT- "to turn"; having individual segments, rather than one rigid bone, allows the torso to turn.

3. **SPONDYL—segment of the spine, vertebra**

    spondylomalacia (SPONDYL-O-malacia) – softening of the vertebrae

    spondylalgia (SPONDYL-algia) – painful condition of the spine

    spondylous (SPONDYL-ous) – pertaining to a vertebra

4. **MYEL—bone marrow, spinal cord**

    myelogenesis (MYEL-O-genesis) – production of bone marrow

    amyelencephalia (*a*-MYEL-ENCEPHAL-ia) – condition of being without brain and spinal cord

    poliomyelitis (POLI-O-MYEL-itis) – inflammation of the spinal cord gray matter

The spinal cord is a bundle of nervous tissue that extends from the brain stem (posterior part of the brain) to the second lumbar vertebra (just above your navel). Because of some resemblance to bone marrow, the name myelin was given to the lipoprotein that coats certain nerve cell structures. We can think of MYELIN- as a base:

5. **MYELIN—myelin, myelin sheath**

    myelinated (MYELIN-ated) – composed of myelin

    myelinolysis (MYELIN-O-lysis) – loosening of myelin sheath, i.e., loss of the myelin sheath

    myelinoclasis (MYELIN-O-clasis) – breakage of myelin sheath, i.e., destruction of the myelin sheath

6. **THORAC—chest, thorax**

    thoracic (THORAC-ic) – pertaining to the chest

    thoracocentesis (THORAC-O-centesis) – puncturing of the chest (cavity)

    thoracomyodynia (THORAC-O-MY-odynia) – painful condition of the muscles of the chest

The Greek term *thorax* originally described a piece of armor that covered the chest. There are twelve thoracic vertebrae in the chest area of the spine. Above these are seven cervical vertebrae; the topmost of these is called the atlas (we mentioned this in a previous chapter), while the second in line is called the axis, and it provides the pivot on which the atlas can rotate:

7. AX—axis, central line

adaxial (*ad*-AX-ial) – pertaining to toward an axis

abaxial (*ab*-AX-ial) – pertaining to away from an axis

We have already met this base previously, but I want to say a little more about it. In antiquity, the term for the axis bone was *axon*; in the 19th century, the term axon was given to the long nerve fibers that project from nerve cells:

AX—axon

axotomy (AX-O-tomy) – surgical cutting of an axon

axolysis (AX-O-lysis) – loosening of an axon, i.e., destruction of an axon

In almost all cases, the base AX- plus the combining vowel "i" denotes an axis, while the same base plus the combining vowel "o" denotes an axon, but note this exception:

axometer (AX-O-meter) – instrument used to measure (or determine) the axis (of an optical lens)

8. STETH—chest

stethomyitis (STETH-O-MY-itis) – inflammation of the muscles of the chest (wall)

stethocyrtometer (STETH-O-CYRT-O-meter) – instrument used to measure the curved (part) of the chest, i.e., instrument used to measure the curvature of the chest

stethoscope (STETH-O-scope) – instrument used to examine the chest

9. PECTOR—chest

pectoralis (PECTOR-alis) – pertaining to the chest

pectoral (PECTOR-al) – pertaining to the chest

pectoralgia (PECTOR-algia) – painful condition of the chest

expectorant (*ex*-PECTOR-ant) – pertaining to out of the chest, i.e., pertaining to promoting the expulsion of phlegm from the chest area

10. MAZ—breast

mazoplasia (MAZ-O-plasia) – surgical reshaping of the breast

tetramazia (TETR-A-MAZ-ia) – condition of the breasts—(having) four of them

Remember, we have already seen the related base MAST- meaning "breast"; it is much more common in compound terms than MAZ-.

11. MAMM—breast

mammary (MAMM-ary) – pertaining to the breast

mammotomy (MAMM-O-tomy) – surgical cutting of the breast

mammectomy (MAMM-ectomy) – surgical removal of the breast

mammilla (MAMM-illa) – small breast, i.e., nipple

12. MAMMILL—nipple

mammillate (MAMMILL-ate) – having nipples, or nipplelike projections

mammillitis (MAMMILL-itis) – inflammation of the nipple

You may also see the alternative spelling MAMILL- for this base. Remember, we saw the base PAPILL- meaning "nipple, papilla" in a previous chapter.

13. COST—rib

intercostal (*inter*-COST-al) – pertaining to between the ribs

costochondral (COST-O-CHONDR-al) – pertaining to the cartilage (attached to the) rib

costiferous (COST-I-FER-ous) – pertaining to bearing ribs

14. STERN—breast bone, sternum

hyposternal (*hypo*-STERN-al) – pertaining to below the sternum

sternocleidomastoidal (STERN-O-CLEID-O-MASTOID-al) – pertaining to the mastoid process, clavicle (collarbone) and sternum

schistosternia (SCHIST-O-STERN-ia) – condition of the sternum (being) split

sternoschisis (STERN-O-schisis) – fission of the sternum

The sternum is the long, flat bone that forms the central portion of the rib cage. It is shaped somewhat like a sword, which is reflected in the vocabulary used to describe it. It is made up of the manubrium, a term derived from MANU- ("hand") meaning "handle," the body, and the xiphoid process, which is a term related to the Greek for "sword":

15. **XIPH—sword**

xiphoid (XIPH-oid) – resembling a sword

You may come across both XIPH- and XIPHOID- as bases meaning the xiphoid process:

XIPH—xiphoid process

XIPHOID—xiphoid process

xiphodynia (XIPH-odynia) – painful condition (in the region of) the xiphoid process

xiphocostal (XIPH-O-COST-al) – pertaining to the ribs and the xiphoid process

xiphoidalgia (XIPHOID-algia) – painful condition (in the region of) the xiphoid process

16. **LUMB—loin**

lumbar (LUMB-ar) – pertaining to the loin

supralumbar (*supra*-LUMB-ar) – pertaining to (the region above) the loin

lumbocostal (LUMB-O-COST-al) – pertaining to the rib and loin (region)

The "loin" is a somewhat imprecise term; it generally indicates the parts of the body below the ribs and above the hip bones; however, in everyday language, it is often used about the genital area. There are five lumbar vertebrae in the spine; below them, five vertebrae are fused into a single bone, the sacrum.

17. **SACR—sacred, holy**

sacral (SACR-al) – pertaining to (something) holy

Why the sacrum bone (literally, a "sacred thing") got its name is unclear, and we will not go into the competing theories about its derivation here. In medical terminology, the base SACR- always refers to the sacrum bone:

SACR—sacrum

sacral (SACR-al) – pertaining to the sacrum

sacrad (SACR-ad) – toward the sacrum

sacrectomy (SACR-ectomy) – surgical removal (of part) of the sacrum

18. **COCCY—cuckoo**

coccycephaly (COCCY-CEPHAL-y) – condition of the head (bearing resemblance to) a cuckoo's (beak), i.e., a malformation in which the head looks like a beak when viewed from the side

The coccyx, or tail bone, is located at the bottom end of the spinal column. It is made up of usually four, but sometimes three or five, small bones fused together. It takes its name from its supposed resemblance to a cuckoo's beak:

COCCY—coccyx, tail bone
COCCYG—coccyx, tail bone

coccyalgia (COCCY-algia) – painful condition of the coccyx

coccygeal (COCCYG-eal) – pertaining to the coccyx

coccygotomy (COCCYG-O-tomy) – surgical cutting of the coccyx

sacrococcygeal (SACR-O-COCCYG-eal) – pertaining to the coccyx and sacrum

Here are some bases that are used in terms describing features associated with bones, including the vertebrae:

19. FOR—to bore, to pierce

imperforate (*im-per*-FOR-ate) – having not through piercing, i.e., lacking a normal opening

transforation (*trans*-FOR-ation) – process of through piercing, i.e., process of piercing through the fetal head to aid delivery

The term imperforate is another example of a *prefix-prefix*-BASE-suffix type. We can approach it just as we have done previously for similar terms; start with the suffix, then add the first prefix, then the second prefix, then add in your base, and add in any words necessary to make good sense. The result here is quite clumsy—"having not through piercing"—but it conveys the meaning accurately and then we can adjust it to make it more elegant if we choose to. The word foramen (plural foramina) is related to the base FOR-; it is the medical term for an opening or perforation in a bone or other structure that allows muscles, nerves, arteries, and veins to pass through. We can think of FORAMIN- as a base:

20. FORAMIN—foramen, opening

foraminal (FORAMIN-al) – pertaining to a foramen

foraminotomy (FORAMIN-O-tomy) – surgical cutting of a foramen (to enlarge it)

foraminiferous (FORAMIN-I-FER-ous) – pertaining to bearing foramina, i.e., pertaining to having foramina

21. ARC—arch, bow

arciform (ARC-I-form) – (shaped) like an arch

arcual (ARC-ual) – pertaining to an arch

In anatomy, an arcus is any structure that resembles an arch or bent bow. Related to ARC- is the base ARCUAT-, meaning "arched" or "bow shaped." Areas of bones, as well as other body structures, may be termed arcuate if they display an arched form.

22. EMIN—standing out, projecting

eminence (EMIN-ence) – state of projecting

An area of bone that is raised higher than the surrounding area may be named an eminence; the arcuate eminence, for example, is a prominent portion of the temporal bone. You may also come across the term in the original Latin form, *eminentia*.

23. PROMIN—standing out, prominent

prominence (PROMIN-ence) – state of being prominent

An area of bone, tissue, or body part that projects beyond a surface may be named a prominence or, using a related term, a promontory; the sacral promontory, for example, is a prominent portion of the first sacral vertebra. You may also come across the term in the original Latin forms, *prominentia* or *promontorium*. There is not a huge difference between an eminence and a prominence.

24. APIC—tip, summit, apex

periapical (*peri*-APIC-al) – pertaining to around the tip

apicoectomy (APIC-O-ectomy) – surgical removal of the tip (of a dental root)

apicolysis (APIC-O-lysis) – surgical separation of the apex (of the lung)

apicostomy (APIC-O-stomy) – making a surgical opening (to reach) the apex (of a dental root)

In anatomy, the apex refers to the tip or extremity of a structure; the sacral apex, for example, is the inferior (i.e., lower down) end of the sacrum.

25. POR—passage, cavity, pore

porous (POR-ous) – full of openings

porencephalitis (POR-ENCEPHAL-itis) – inflammation of the brain (with the formation of) cavities (within it)

osteoporosis (OSTE-O-POR-osis) – abnormal condition of porous bone, i.e., condition of bones that are more porous than solid

porotomy (POR-O-tomy) – surgical cutting (to enlarge a body) passage

The brain and spinal cord, enclosed within the skull and vertebral column, together make up the central nervous system. We have already looked at many of the terms associated with them; here are some bases associated with the peripheral nervous system that is made up of the cranial and spinal nerves, and their branches. The peripheral nervous system is responsible for communication between the central nervous system and the rest of the body:

26. NEUR—nerve, nervous system, tendon

neurology (NEUR-O-logy) – study of the nervous system

neurectopia (NEUR-*ec*-TOP-ia) – condition of outside the (correct) position nerve, i.e., condition of a displacement of a nerve

odontoneuralgia (ODONT-O-NEUR-algia) – painful condition of the nerves (due to a decaying) tooth

In neurectopia, we have another term where a base precedes the prefix; we can use exactly the same method that we used for adenectopy to build up the term. Sometimes, the base NEUR- can be a little tricky. It can, for example, indicate a specific nerve:

neurochorioretinitis (NEUR-O-CHORI-O-RETIN-itis) – inflammation of the retina, choroid, and optic nerve

It can also have the meaning "nerve" in the sense of emotion or feeling, as in the sayings "you're getting on my nerves," or "he's just a bag of nerves." Therefore, a neurosis,

neurosis (NEUR-osis) – abnormal condition of the nerves

may be a psychological disorder marked by anxiety, or a state of nervousness, as well as a functional condition affecting the nerves or nervous system. In addition, while NEUR- almost always has the meaning "nerve" or "nervous system," occasionally the meaning "tendon" shows up; an aponeurosis, for example, has nothing at all to do with the types of neurosis we have just looked at, it is actually a tendonlike structure that attaches muscles to bones.

27. NERV—nerve

abnerval (*ab*-NERV-al) – away from a nerve

adnerval (*ad*-NERV-al) – near a nerve

While the word nerve is exceedingly common in anatomical vocabulary, the base NERV- rarely appears in medical compound terms.

There are twelve pairs of cranial nerves; each pair either receives sensory information from the body or sends motor information to the brain:

28. SENS—to feel, to perceive, sense
SENT—to feel, to perceive, sense

sensory (SENS-ory) – having the function of feeling or perception

hemisensory (HEMI-SENS-ory) – having the function of feeling in half (the body), i.e., loss of feeling on one side of the body

sentience (SENT-I-ence) – state of feeling, i.e., ability to perceive stimuli

29. MOT—to move, movement

motor (MOT-or) – thing that moves or (causes) movement

motile (MOT-ile) – able to move

oculomotor (OCUL-O-MOT-or) – thing that moves the eye

There are thirty-one pairs of spinal nerves that arise from the spinal cord; each of these nerves has both sensory and motor nerve roots that connect to the cord:

30. RHIZ—root
-RRHIZ—root

rhizoid (RHIZ-oid) – resembling a root

rhizotomy (RHIZ-O-tomy) – surgical cutting of a (spinal nerve) root

rhizomeningomyelitis (RHIZ-O-MENING-O-MYEL-itis) – inflammation of the spinal cord, meninges, and (spinal nerve) roots

polyrrhizal (POLY-RRHIZ-al) – pertaining to roots—many of them

The form -RRHIZ- only occurs in the middle of a term, never at the beginning.

31. RADIC—root

radicotomy (RADIC-O-tomy) – surgical cutting of a (spinal nerve) root

radicula (RADIC-ula) – small root, i.e., a radicle

The term radicula is used about the spinal nerve roots; we can think of RADICUL- as a base:

32. RADICUL—spinal nerve root, radicle

radicular (RADICUL-ar) – pertaining to a radicle

radiculalgia (RADICUL-algia) – painful condition of the (sensory) spinal nerve roots

radiculomyelopathy (RADICUL-O-MYEL-O-pathy) – disease of the spinal cord and the spinal nerve roots

Within the peripheral nervous system, the autonomic nervous system controls involuntary movement, while the somatic (we have seen SOMAT-ic previously) nervous system controls voluntary movement:

33. AUT—self

autodermic (AUT-O-DERM-ic) – pertaining to the skin of oneself, i.e., pertaining to one's own skin for use in skin grafts

autophilia (AUT-O-philia) – condition of attraction to oneself, i.e., condition of narcissism (remember the story of Echo and Narcissus)

autophobia (AUT-O-phobia) – abnormal fear of oneself, i.e., fear of being isolated

34. NOM—law, custom

nomogenesis (NOM-O-genesis) – production (according to) law, i.e., evolution according to predetermined law and not through chance

nomotopic (NOM-O-TOP-ic) – pertaining to the place (that is) customary, i.e., pertaining to the usual or normal place

autonomic (AUT-O-NOM-ic) – pertaining to the laws of oneself, i.e., pertaining to not being controlled by external forces

All neural tissue of the nervous system is made up of neurons that generate and conduct electrical impulses, and neuroglia, cells that perform a range of functions that help neurons do their work. The neuroglia got their name because they were thought of as the glue that held the nervous system together:

35. GLI—glue

You will probably never come across this base in any context other than glial or neuroglial cells (glia and neuroglia refer to the same type of cells):

GLI—glia, neuroglia

glioma (GLI-oma) – tumor (derived from) glia

microglial (MICR-O-GLI-al) – pertaining to glia (that are) small

36. LEMM—cover, sheath

neurilemmitis (NEUR-I-LEMM-itis) – inflammation of the sheath of a nerve, i.e., inflammation of the neurilemma

myolemmal (MY-O-LEMM-al) – pertaining to the sheath of a muscle (fiber), i.e., pertaining to a myolemma

trichilemmoma (TRICH-I-LEMM-oma) – tumor (derived from the) sheath of a hair (follicle)

The neurilemma (or sometimes neurolemma) is the protective sheath that surrounds the nerve axon.

37. GANGLI—swelling, knot

You will come across this base in two contexts, associated with clusters of nerve cells or nerve cell bodies, and with fluid-filled swellings that develop around tendons. The structure, in both cases, is termed a ganglion (plural ganglia):

GANGLI—ganglion
GANGLION—ganglion

ganglioneuroma (GANGLI-O-NEUR-oma) – tumor of nerve (cell) ganglia
gangliate (GANGLI-ate) – having ganglia
ganglionectomy (GANGLION-ectomy) – surgical removal of a ganglion

SOME MORE THINGS TO LEARN

Here are some more bases related to movement, muscles, tendons, ligaments, and associated structures:

38. THEC—cover, sheath

thecal (THEC-al) – pertaining to a sheath (especially a tendon sheath)
thecitis (THEC-itis) – inflammation of a sheath (of a tendon)
intrathecal (*intra*-THEC-al) – pertaining to within a sheath

The term theca often, but not always, refers to the sheath or covering of a tendon; intrathecal may refer to the space between the spinal cord and its protective sheath.

39. FIBR—fiber, filament

fibril (FIBR-il) – small fiber, or a small (component of a) fiber
fibrilla (FIBR-illa) – small fiber, or a small (component of a) fiber
fibromyalgia (FIBR-O-MY-algia) – painful condition of the muscle fibers
fibroma (FIBR-oma) – tumor (derived from) fibrous (tissue)
fibrin (FIBR-in) – substance (composed of) filaments (containing protein), i.e., a fibrous protein involved in blood clotting

Fibers are generally long, slender threads or filaments of tissue, especially connective tissue, or certain specialized cells of muscles and nerves. Fibrin is a fibrous protein that is important in blood clotting, produced by the action of a specific enzyme on the glycoprotein (protein containing carbohydrate) fibrinogen; we can think of FIBRIN- as a base:

40. FIBRIN—fibrin

fibrinous (FIBRIN-ous) – pertaining to fibrin

fibrinogenesis (FIBRIN-O-genesis) – production of fibrin

fibrinogenopenia (FIBRIN-O-GEN-O-penia) – deficiency of that which produces fibrin, i.e., deficiency of fibrinogen

41. IN—fiber

inogenesis (IN-O-genesis) – production of fibrous tissue

inosclerosis (IN-O-SCLER-osis) – abnormal hardening (due to) fibrous tissue

This base has largely been replaced by FIBR-, but you may still come across it. It is almost always followed by the combining vowel "o," so you should be able to easily distinguish it from the prefix *in*-.

42. BURS—sac, pouch, bursa

bursate (BURS-ate) – having a sac(-like receptacle)

bursitis (BURS-itis) – inflammation of a bursa

bursectomy (BURS-ectomy) – surgical removal of a bursa

A bursa is a small sac filled with fluid, often between parts that rub against each other.

43. PONT—bridge

pontic (PONT-ic) – pertaining to a bridge

In dentistry, a pontic is a false tooth that bridges a gap. In anatomy, a pons is a bridge of tissue that connects two parts of a structure or organ:

PONT—pons

pontine (PONT-ine) – pertaining to a pons

cerebellopontine (CEREBELL-O-PONT-ine) – pertaining to the (brainstem) pons and the cerebellum

ponticulus (PONT-I-culus) – a small pons

44. KINE—to move, movement
KINES—movement
KINET—movement

adipokinesis (ADIP-O-KINE-sis) – process of movement of fat (within the body)

eukinesia (*eu*-KINES-ia) – condition of normal movement

kinesophobia (KINES-O-phobia) – abnormal fear of movement

bradykinetic (BRADY-KINET-ic) – pertaining to moving slowly

If you come across any of these bases beginning with a "c" in place of a "k," they generally refer to the movement of motion pictures.

45. TACT—(i) to touch, touching: (ii) order, arrangement
TAX—order, arrangement
TAXI—order, arrangement

barotactic (BAR-O-TACT-ic) – pertaining to arrangement (in response to) pressure, i.e., pertaining to reaction of bodily tissues to changes in pressure

ataxia (*a*-TAX-ia) – condition of without order, i.e., condition of lack of co-ordination of the muscles

ataxiaphasia (*a*-TAXI-A-PHAS-ia) – condition of speech without order, i.e., condition of inability to form connected sentences

We have already looked at the meanings "to touch, touching" for the base TACT- in an earlier chapter. Note that the term ataxiaphasia is unusual in that the prefix does not relate to the ultimate base.

46. CLON—violent motion, spasm

clonic (CLON-ic) – pertaining to violent motion (of a muscle), i.e., pertaining to rapid contraction and relaxation of a muscle

logoclonia (LOG-O-CLON-ia) – condition of spasmodic (repetition of) words

The term clonus is applied to a muscular spasm that involves rapid contraction and relaxation.

47. TROPH—nourishment, nutrition

atrophy (*a*-TROPH-y) – condition of non-nourishment, i.e., condition of wasting

amyotrophia (*a*-MY-O-TROPH-ia) – condition of non-nourishment of muscles, i.e., condition of wasting of the muscles

dystrophia (*dys*-TROPH-ia) – condition of abnormal nourishment, i.e., condition of progressive weakness due to lack of nourishment

trophopathy (TROPH-O-pathy) – disease (due to) nutritional (causes)

The combinations *a*-TROPH-ia, *a*-TROPH-y and *dys*-TROPH-ia, *dys*-TROPH-y are so common that we can add atrophia, atrophy and dystrophia, dystrophy to our list of compound suffixes. Like the term asthenia that we saw previously, they are actually prefix, base, and suffix combinations.

1. -atrophia, -atrophy	wasting
2. -dystrophia, -dystrophy	weakness

Chapter 13

LUNGS

SUFFIXES

1. -ase	enzyme (chemistry)
2. -ol	alcohol (chemistry)
3. -one	ketone (chemistry)
4. -ose	sugar (chemistry)
5. -ulent	full of

Sometimes, you will come across suffixes from chemistry or biochemistry that indicate certain types of compounds. We will only look at the more common ones.

BASES

1. **HAL—(i) to breathe, breath: (ii) salt**
   HALIT—breath

   inhalation (*in*-HAL-ation) – process of in breathing

   exhalation (*ex*-HAL-ation) – process of out breathing

halitosis (HALIT-osis) – abnormal condition of the breath, i.e., condition of foul-smelling breath

halophilic (HAL-O-PHIL-ic) – pertaining to having an affinity for salt, i.e., pertaining to needing a high salt concentration to survive

Remember, we have already met the base SPIR- ("to breathe") that gives us terms such as respiratory, respiration, inspiration, and expiration. You are much more likely to come across the base HAL- meaning "to breathe, breath" than "salt"; the two meanings come from two unrelated Latin words, but it is easy to confuse the two and, as always, you will have to rely on context to help you decide on the correct meaning.

2. **VENTIL—to fan, to set air in motion**

ventilate (VENTIL-ate) – to cause air to be set in motion, i.e., to move gases in and out of the lungs

hyperventilation (*hyper*-VENTIL-ation) – process of more than normal movement of air (in the lungs), i.e., process of extremely rapid or deep breathing leading to increased oxygen in the blood

hypoventilation (*hypo*-VENTIL-ation) – process of less than normal movement of air (in the lungs), i.e., process of extremely slow or shallow breathing leading to decreased oxygen in the blood

3. **PNE—to breathe, breath**

apneic (*a*-PNE-ic) – pertaining to without breathing, i.e., pertaining to momentary suspension of breathing

tachypneic (TACHY-PNE-ic) – pertaining to breathing (that is) fast

dyspneic (*dys*-PNE-ic) – pertaining to breathing (that is) difficult

You will very likely come across the form PNEa (or sometimes PNOEa), meaning "breathing" or "respiration." Like AGRa, which we saw previously, it is actually closer to an unmodified Greek noun than it is to a BASE-suffix combination. It is probably better to think of it as one of the compound suffixes:

bradypnea (BRADY-pnea) – breathing that is slow

eupnea (*eu*-pnea) – breathing that is normal

hyperpnea (*hyper*-pnea) – breathing that is more than normal, i.e., breathing that is extremely rapid or deep

Notice how treating -pnea as a compound suffix means we can have terms that seem to have no base. We know that this cannot really be so, since it is the base that carries the basic meaning and sense of the term.

4. TRACH—rough

trachyphonia (TRACH-Y-PHON-ia) – condition of the voice that is rough

You will not find this base used a lot in medical terminology, but the ancient medics used it to refer to the "rough artery," meaning the windpipe; all arteries were believed to carry air, only the windpipe was the "rough artery," all others were "smooth arteries." In later vocabulary, the windpipe was given the name trachea. We can think of TRACHE- as a base:

5. TRACHE—windpipe, trachea

tracheoschisis (TRACHE-O-schisis) – fissure into the trachea

tracheotomy (TRACHE-O-tomy) – surgical cutting of the trachea

tracheopharyngeal (TRACHE-O-PHARYNG-eal) – pertaining to the pharynx and trachea

The trachea is the airway below the larynx. A column of C-shaped rings of cartilage provide support for the trachea, so that it does not collapse when air is drawn through it. Be careful not to confuse this base with TRACHEL-, "neck."

6. BRONCH—bronchus, airway

bronchoedema (BRONCH-O-edema) – swelling of the bronchi (membranes)

bronchial (BRONCH-ial) – pertaining to the bronchi

bronchostenosis (BRONCH-O-stenosis) – narrowing of a bronchus

bronchiole (BRONCH-I-ole) – small bronchus

The inferior part of the trachea (windpipe) divides into two smaller airways, the left primary bronchus and the right primary bronchus (plural bronchi). As each primary bronchus enters a lung, it subdivides into secondary and then tertiary bronchi (also called lobar and segmental bronchi), and finally into small bronchi called bronchioles. We can think of BRONCHIOL- as a base:

7. BRONCHIOL—bronchiole

bronchiolitis (BRONCHIOL-itis) – inflammation of the bronchioles

bronchiolectasis (BRONCHIOL-ectasis) – dilation of the bronchioles

While the bronchi contain some cartilage, the bronchioles contain no cartilage at all. The bronchioles terminate in alveoli, hollow air sacs lined with the cells in which the gas exchanges associated with respiration occur. The term alveolus (plural alveoli) is used about several other cavitylike structures in the body in addition to the respiratory alveoli; the wall of the stomach is lined with alveoli, and the hollow in which a tooth sits is termed an alveolus.

8. **ALVEOL—hollow, cavity, socket, alveolus**

    alveolalgia (ALVEOL-algia) – painful condition of (tooth) socket

    alveolate (ALVEOL-ate) – having alveoli

    alveolitis (ALVEOL-itis) – inflammation of the alveoli

9. **AER—air, gas**

    aerosis (AER-osis) – abnormal condition of gas or air (in tissues or organs)

    anaerogenic (*an*-AER-O-genic) – producing not gas, i.e., not producing gas

    aerodontalgia (AER-ODONT-algia) – painful condition of a tooth (due to) air (pressure)

10. **PNEUM—(i) air, gas: (ii) lung**
    PNEUMAT—air, gas

    pneumarthrosis (PNEUM-ARTHR-osis) – abnormal condition of a joint (containing) air or gas

    pneumocephalic (PNEUM-O-CEPHAL-ic) – pertaining to the cranium (containing) air or gas

    pneumohypodermal (PNEUM-O-*hypo*-DERM-al) – pertaining to below the skin air or gas, i.e., pertaining to subcutaneous air or gas in the tissues

    pneumatics (PNEUMAT-ics) – science of (properties of) air and gas

Pneumohypodermal is another example of a term where a base precedes a prefix. Use the same method as previously—leave the base that precedes the prefix till last, treat the remaining *prefix*-BASE-suffix in the normal manner (always start with the suffix, then add the prefix, and then add in your base) and then add in the other base last.

11. **PNEUM—(i) lung: (ii) air, gas**
    PNEUMON—lung

    apneumia (*a*-PNEUM-ia) – condition of (being) without lungs

    pneumomalacia (PNEUM-O-malacia) – softening of lung (tissue)

    pneumomelanosis (PNEUM-O-MELAN-osis) – condition of blackening of lung (tissue)

    pneumonectomy (PNEUMON-ectomy) – surgical removal of a lung

    pneumonia (PNEUMON-ia) – condition of the lungs

While the ancient Greek words for "air" and "lung" are different (but related), they each have the base PNEUM-. Sometimes it is easy to distinguish which meaning is intended; the PNEUM- in pneumomalacia, for example, must refer to "lung"; however, in apneumia, it is not so clear. You will have to hope that context will help you.

12. PULM—lung
PULMON—lung

pulmograph (PULM-O-graph) – instrument used to record lung (function)

pulmonary (PULMON-ary) – pertaining to the lung

pulmonectomy (PULMON-ectomy) – surgical removal of a lung

bronchopulmonary (BRONCH-O-PULMON-ary) – pertaining to the lungs and bronchi

13. PLEUR—rib, side, pleura

pleurapophyseal (PLEUR-*apo*-PHYS-eal) – pertaining to an outgrowth (on a) rib

pleurocentral (PLEUR-O-CENTR-al) – pertaining to (between) the center and the side (of the body), i.e., pertaining to one lateral half of the body

pleuritis (PLEUR-itis) – inflammation of the pleura

pleural (PLEUR-al) – pertaining to the pleura

pleuroclysis (PLEUR-O-clysis) – irrigation of the pleura (and pleural cavity)

Each lung is surrounded by a thin membrane called a pleura (plural pleurae). While this base does have other meanings, "rib" and "side," it most often refers to the pleurae that enclose the lungs, or to related membranes in the chest area. Remember we talked about apophysis, an "outgrowth (of bone)" earlier; the term pleuroapophyseal is another instance of a term in which a base precedes a suffix, but we can use exactly the same method as before for building it up.

14. TEL—completion, end
TELE—completion, end

atelectasis (*a*-TEL-ectasis) – dilation (that is) not complete, i.e., incomplete dilation of a lung

atelencephalia (*a*-TEL-ENCEPHAL-ia) – condition of the brain with non-complete (development)

bradyteleokinesis (BRADY-TELE-O-KINE-sis) – process of movement (in which) completion is slow, i.e., process of movement suddenly halted before conclusion, then completed slowly

Atelectasis is commonly known as a collapsed lung. Note that the term atelencephalia is unusual in that the prefix does not relate to the ultimate base.

15. BOL—to throw, to put

anabolic (*ana*-BOL-ic) – pertaining to up throwing, i.e., pertaining to building up

catabolic (*cata*-BOL-ic) – pertaining to down throwing, i.e., pertaining to breaking down metabolism (*meta*-BOL-ism) – condition of change (in) throwing, i.e., condition of change or transition

The literal definitions here are pretty awkward but you get the idea. Metabolism is the process by which the body converts what you eat and drink into energy. During the anabolism phase of metabolism, chemical reactions build small molecules up into large molecules; during catabolism, chemical reactions break large molecules down into small molecules. More specifically, respiratory metabolism involves the exchange of respiratory gases in the lungs, the oxidation of foodstuffs, and the production of carbon dioxide.

16. OX—(i) acute, sharp, pointed, acid-tasting: (ii) oxygen
OXY—(i) acute, sharp, pointed, acid-tasting: (ii) oxygen

oxyblepsia (OXY-blepsia) – condition of sight that is sharp, i.e., condition of sharp-sightedness

oxycephalia (OXY-CEPHAL-ia) – condition of the head (being) pointed

oxypathia (OXY-pathia) – disease that is acute

hyperoxia (*hyper*-OX-ia) – condition of more than normal oxygen (in the blood and tissues)

The gas oxygen got its name because it was believed, wrongly, that it was an essential element in the formation of all acids.

17. CAPN—(i) smoke: (ii) carbon dioxide

capnomania (CAPN-O-mania) – compulsion to smoke (tobacco products)

capnogram (CAPN-O-gram) – record of (exhaled) carbon dioxide

hypercapnia (*hyper*-CAPN-ia) – condition of more than normal carbon dioxide (in the blood)

Here are four bases that can be found in medical terms related to respiratory diseases:

18. CONI—dust

coniosis (CONI-osis) – condition (caused by) dust

dermatoconiosis (DERMAT-O-CONI-osis) – condition (caused by) dust (affecting) the skin

pneumoconiosis (PNEUM-O-CONI-osis) – condition (caused by) dust (affecting) the lungs

19. SILIC—quartz, silica

silicosis (SILIC-osis) – abnormal condition (caused by) silica, i.e., a respiratory condition resulting from the inhalation of silica dust silicotuberculosis (SILIC-O-TUBERCUL-osis) – abnormal condition of the tubercles and abnormal condition (caused by) silica, i.e., silicosis complicated by tuberculosis (disease caused by the bacterium *Mycobacterium tuberculosis*)

The term pneumonoultramicroscopicsilicovolcanoconiosis is the longest medical term in a dictionary, but it was really just created to get that distinction. This huge term really does not mean much more than silicosis; it is a respiratory condition resulting from the inhalation of very fine silica dust and other particles.

20. CALC—limestone, calcium, pebble

calcification (CALC-I-fication) – process of producing calcium (salts), i.e., the deposition of calcium salts in body tissues

calcipenia (CALC-I-penia) – deficiency of calcium (in the body)

calcicosis (CALC-ic-osis) – abnormal condition pertaining to limestone, i.e., a respiratory condition resulting from the inhalation of limestone dust

calculus (CALC-ulus) – small pebble

The term calcicosis has two suffixes, but we can use the method seen previously. Make a single suffix from the two, starting with the ultimate (last) one; this tells us whether our compound term is a noun, adjective, or verb. Then proceed as normal. In medical terminology, a calculus (plural calculi) is a compact mass of material, usually mineral salts, formed in the body; commonly called a stone, it might form in the kidneys, bladder, or gallbladder. We get the mathematical terms "calculus" and "calculation" from this base because small pebbles were originally used as counters.

21. ANTHRAC—(i) coal, charcoal: (ii) carbuncle

anthracosilicosis (ANTHRAC-O-SILIC-osis) – abnormal condition (caused by) silica and coal, i.e., a respiratory condition resulting from the inhalation of silica and coal dusts

anthracia (ANTHRAC-ia) – condition (characterized by) carbuncles

Anthrax is an acute infection caused by the bacterium *Bacillus anthracis*; the disease and the bacterium got their name from the coal-black sores that are characteristic of the infection.

22. CARB—coal, carbon

carbuncle (CARB-uncle) – small (live) coal, i.e., a fiery-red abscess

carbometry (CARB-O-metry) – process of measuring (exhaled) carbon (dioxide)

The similarity between a red-hot piece of coal and a fiery-red abscess had already been observed before the time of Galen. Carbon compounds are central to the process of respiration and respiratory metabolism.

23. TUSS—cough

tussigenic (TUSS-I-genic) – producing a cough

tussive (TUSS-ive) – pertaining to a cough

24. PY—pus

empyema (*em*-PY-ema) – condition of inward pus, i.e., condition of pus in the lungs or thoracic cavity

dacryopyorrhea (DACRY-O-PY-O-rrhea) – discharge of pus (within) the tears

tracheopyosis (TRACHE-O-PY-osis) – abnormal condition of pus in the trachea

Be careful not to confuse empyema with emphysema (*em*-PHYS-ema); literally a "condition of inward inflation," pulmonary emphysema is a condition in which the alveoli are enlarged, thus trapping air in the lungs and making full expiration difficult.

25. PUR—pus

puromucous (PUR-O-MUC-ous) – pertaining to, or full of, mucus and pus

purulent (PUR-ulent) – full of pus

SOME MORE THINGS TO LEARN

Here is the compound suffix we saw in this chapter:

1. -pnea	breathing, respiration

We have also seen some bases in this chapter that are used about chemical elements and compounds; here are some more to learn, as well as the bases for some common substances. These are mostly bases that you could not be expected to guess; for example, SIDER- meaning "iron." If you come across bases such as FLUOR- or ALUMIN-, you should be able to figure out the meaning.

26. ACET—(i) sour, vinegar: (ii) acetic acid (derivatives)

acetic (ACET-ic) – pertaining to vinegar

acetous (ACET-ous) – like vinegar

acetify (ACET-I-fy) – to make vinegar

acetone (ACET-one) – ketone of acetic acid

27. ACID—sour, acid (i.e., low pH)

acidophilic (ACID-O-PHIL-ic) – pertaining to having an affinity for acids, i.e., pertaining to cells or tissues that have an affinity for acid dyes and stains

acidosis (ACID-osis) – abnormal condition of (increased) acidity (in the blood and tissues)

hyperacidity (*hyper*-ACID-ity) – condition of more than normal acidity

The term alkali, denoting substances at the opposite end of the pH scale to acid, comes from the Arabic word *al-qali*, meaning soda-ash. In many languages, the element that we know as potassium in English is called kalium, a term related to alkali; this is why potassium has the chemical symbol K. Similarly, the alkaline element that English calls sodium is known as natrium in many other languages, and this is why it has the chemical symbol Na.

28. HYDR—water, watery fluid

hydrophobia (HYDR-O-phobia) – abnormal fear of water

hydrocephalic (HYDR-O-CEPHAL-ic) – pertaining to a brain (affected by) water, i.e., pertaining to an abnormal accumulation of fluid within the brain, sometimes called water on the brain in everyday language

anhydrous (*an*-HYDR-ous) – pertaining to without water

Remember, we have also seen the base AQU-, AQUE- meaning "water, watery fluid."

29. KALI—potassium

kaliopenia (KALI-O-penia) – deficiency of potassium (in the body)

30. NATR—sodium

natriferic (NATR-I-FER-ic) – pertaining to carrying sodium, i.e., pertaining to sodium transport in the body

31. GLUC—sweet, sugar
GLYC—sweet, sugar

glucolysis (GLUC-O-lysis) – loosening of sugar, i.e., conversion of sugar (usually glucose) to lactic acid

cytoglucopenia (CYT-O-GLUC-O-penia) – deficiency of sugar (glucose) within the cells

glycorrhea (GLYC-O-rrhea) – discharge of sugar, i.e., excretion of sugar from the body, usually in the urine

glycol (GLYC-ol) – alcohol (that is) sweet, a common name for both ethylene glycol and propylene glycol

32. SACCHAR—sweet, sugar

saccharic (SACCHAR-ic) – pertaining to sugar

saccharimeter (SACCHAR-I-meter) – instrument used to measure sugar (in a solution)

sacchariferous (SACCHAR-I-FER-ous) – pertaining to producing sugar

33. AMYL—starch

amyloid (AMYL-oid) – resembling starch

amylogenesis (AMYL-O-genesis) – production of starch

amylorrhea (AMYL-O-rrhea) – discharge of (undigested) starch

amylase (AMYL-ase) – enzyme (that breaks down) starch

The term amyloid is also used about a number of insoluble and irregularly formed protein compounds that may form in the body; the condition amyloidosis is characterized by the accumulation of amyloids in organs and tissues, preventing proper functioning.

34. SIDER—iron

siderophilous (SIDER-O-PHIL-ous) – pertaining to having an affinity for iron, i.e., pertaining to absorbing iron in the body

siderodermatic (SIDER-O-DERMAT-ic) – pertaining to skin (that is) iron (oxide, i.e., rust) colored, i.e., pertaining to a brownish discoloration on the skin due to an iron-complex deposit

siderogenous (SIDER-O-genous) – producing iron

35. FERR—iron

ferrotherapy (FERR-O-therapy) – treatment (of disease) using iron

ferrous (FERR-ous) – pertaining to iron

ferrometer (FERR-O-meter) – instrument used to measure (the quantity of) iron (in the blood)

36. THI—sulfur

thiogenic (THI-O-genic) – producing sulfur

You will mostly see SULF- or SULPH- as the base meaning sulfur, but occasionally you may come across THI-, which derives from the ancient Greek word for sulfur.

37. ARGYR—silver

argyria (ARGYR-ia) – condition of silver (poisoning)

argyrophilic (ARGYR-O-PHIL-ic) – pertaining to having an affinity for silver, i.e., pertaining to tissues that can bind to silver ions, which can then be reduced to a dark stain

38. ARGENT—silver

argentophilic (ARGENT-O-PHIL-ic) – pertaining to having an affinity for silver, i.e., pertaining to tissues that can bind to silver ions, which can then be reduced to a dark stain

39. CHRYS—gold

chrysotherapy (CHRYS-O-therapy) – treatment (of disease) with gold (salts)

chrysiasis (CHRYS-iasis) – abnormal condition (due to) gold, i.e., condition of skin discoloration due to therapy using gold salts

40. AUR—gold

aurotherapy (AUR-O-therapy) – treatment (of disease) with gold (salts)

aurochromodermatic (AUR-O-CHROM-O-DERMAT-ic) – pertaining to skin that is colored (due to) gold, i.e., pertaining to skin discoloration due to therapy using gold salts

Be careful not to confuse this base with AUR- meaning "ear."

41. GALACT—milk

galactorrhea (GALACT-O-rrhea) – flow of milk, i.e., abnormal flow not associated with nursing an infant

galactophorous (GALACT-O-PHOR-ous) – pertaining to carrying milk, i.e., pertaining to the milk ducts

oligogalactia (OLIG-O-GALACT-ia) – condition of milk (being) scanty, i.e., condition of scant secretion of milk in a nursing mother

42. LACT—milk

lactiferous (LACT-I-FER-ous) – pertaining to producing milk

lactation (LACT-ation) – process (of secretion) of milk

lactose (LACT-ose) – sugar (found in) milk

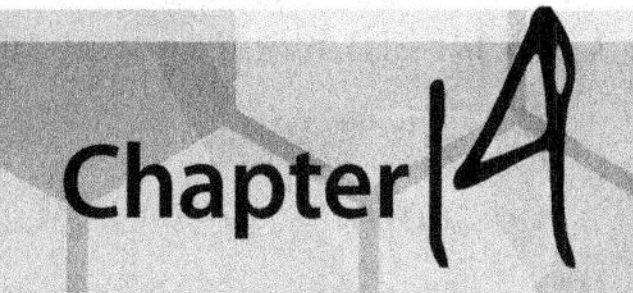

HEART, BLOOD, LYMPH, AND SPLEEN

SUFFIXES

1. -ative	pertaining to, tending to

BASES

1. **CARD—(i) heart: (ii) cardia (upper portion of the stomach)**
   CARDI—(i) heart: (ii) cardia (upper portion of the stomach)

   bradycardic (BRADY-CARD-ic) – pertaining to heart (rate that is abnormally) slow

   myocardial (MY-O-CARDI-al) – pertaining to the heart muscle

   cardioplegia (CARDI-O-plegia) – paralysis of the heart

   cardiectomy (CARDI-ectomy) – surgical removal of the cardia (upper portion of the stomach)

Ancient physicians used the term cardia (or kardia) about the heart and about the upper part of the stomach closest to the heart. You are more likely to come across this base with the meaning "heart" but, as always, you have to use common sense and decide from context which meaning of the two is the most suitable.

2. **CORD—(i) heart: (ii) cord**
   cordate (CORD-ate) – having the shape of a heart
   postcordial (*post*-CORD-ial) – pertaining to behind the heart
   cordectomy (CORD-ectomy) – surgical removal of (an anatomical) cord

Medical terminology uses the base CARDI- to mean "heart" much more frequently than this base. Likewise, you will probably see the base CHORD- meaning "cord," as in "vocal cord," more often, but do be aware that CORD- can also have this meaning.

3. **ATRI—chamber, entrance hall**
   atrial (ATRI-al) – pertaining to a chamber

Several chambers or cavities within the body are termed atria (singular atrium); there are atria within the ear, lung, and brain, but you are most likely to come across the ones in the heart. The heart is divided into four chambers; each of the two larger lower chambers is called a ventricle, while each upper chamber is called an atrium:

ATRI—atrium (chamber of the heart)
interatrial (*inter*-ATRI-al) – pertaining to between the atria
atriomegaly (ATRI-O-megaly) – enlargement of the atrium
atriotomy (ATRI-O-tomy) – surgical cutting of an atrium

We have met the base VENTR- previously, meaning "front, abdomen, belly." A ventricle, VENTR-I-cle, is literally a "small belly," in the sense of a chamber or cavity. Like the atria, there are ventricles in areas of the body other than the heart, such as the brain and larynx. We can think of VENTRICUL- as a base:

4. **VENTRICUL—ventricle**
   ventricular (VENTRICUL-ar) – pertaining to a ventricle
   ventriculitis (VENTRICUL-itis) – inflammation of a ventricle (of the brain)
   ventriculoplasty (VENTRICUL-O-plasty) – surgical reshaping (repair) of a ventricle (of the heart)

Remember, we came across the term auricle, meaning "little ear, outer ear," in an earlier chapter, but we also noted that it could be used about the ear-shaped projections within the heart. Very occasionally, you may find the term auricle used as an alternative name for atrium, as in auriculoventricular, a synonym for atrioventricular.

5. **VALV—valve**
   VALVUL—valve

   valval (VALV-al) – pertaining to a valve

   valvoplasty (VALV-O-plasty) – surgical reshaping of a valve

   cardiovalvulitis (CARDI-O-VALVUL-itis) – inflammation of a valve of the heart

In the body, valves are folds of membrane or tissue that act like flaps restricting or directing the flow of bodily fluids. Flow of blood through the heart is controlled by four valves; the pulmonary valve, the tricuspid valve, the mitral valve, and the aortic valve.

6. **CUSP—point, tip**

   cuspid (CUSP-id) – having a point or tip

In dentistry, a cusp is one of the elevated points on the chewing surface of a tooth; in anatomy, cusp generally refers to one of the pointed flaps that make up a heart valve:

CUSP—cusp

bicuspid (BI-CUSP-id) – having cusps—two of them

tricuspid (TRI-CUSP-id) – having cusps—three of them

multicuspid (MULTI-CUSP-id) – having cusps—many of them

The term multicuspid is usually used about molar teeth that have three or more cusps. The tricuspid valve of the heart has three cusps, while the mitral valve has two cusps; an alternative name for the mitral valve is the bicuspid valve. The term mitral comes from the base MITR- meaning "turban" or "headband," with the meaning, specifically, like a bishop's miter (a tall hat with two points). You will probably only ever come across the base MITR- in this context.

7. **AORT—artery, aorta**

   aortostenosis (AORT-O-stenosis) – narrowing of the aorta

   aortorrhaphy (AORT-O-rrhaphy) – surgical suture of the aorta

Originally meaning any large artery, the term aorta and the base AORT- now refer to the main artery of the body that originates in the left ventricle and extends downward toward the abdomen.

8. **VAS—vessel**

   vasoneuropathy (VAS-O-NEUR-O-pathy) – disease of the nerves and (blood) vessels vasohypertonic (VAS-O-*hyper*-TON-ic) – pertaining to above normal tension of a (blood) vessel

vasculum (VAS-culum) – small (blood) vessel

Vasohypertonic is another example of a term in which a base precedes a prefix; remember, leave the base that precedes the prefix till last, treat the remaining *prefix*-BASE-suffix in the normal manner (always start with the suffix, then add the prefix, and then add in your base) and then add in the other base last. The base VAS- can mean a vessel that carries any fluid, but it almost always indicates a blood vessel. The noun vas can be used about a vessel, duct, or canal that carries liquid, including lymph and semen, as well as blood:

VAS—vas

vasal (VAS-al) – pertaining to a vas

vasectomy (VAS-ectomy) – surgical removal (of a section) of the vas (deferens), i.e., excision of the sperm duct

We can also think of VASCUL- as a base; in practice, it does not really differ from the base VAS- meaning "vessel":

9. VASCUL—vessel

vasculogenesis (VASCUL-O-genesis) – production of (blood) vessels

vasculature (VASCUL-ature) – system composed of (blood) vessels

10. ANGI—vessel

angiocarditis (ANGI-O-CARD-itis) – inflammation of the heart and (blood) vessels

angiectopia (ANGI-ectopia) – displacement of a (blood) vessel

cardioangiology (CARDI-O-ANGI-O-logy) – study of the (blood) vessels and the heart

11. ARTER—artery
ARTERI—artery

arteritis (ARTER-itis) – inflammation of an artery

arteriole (ARTERI-ole) – a small artery

arteriopathy (ARTERI-O-pathy) – disease of the arteries

12. ANEURYSM—dilation

This base is really a compound of the prefix *ana*-, "up," and the base EURY- meaning "wide," but the two were already put together in ancient Greek; we will treat it here as a single base meaning "dilation," i.e., a widening up of something. It generally has the specific meaning of a dilation of an artery:

ANEURYSM—dilation of an artery, aneurysm

aneurysmal (ANEURYSM-al) – pertaining to an aneurysm

aneurysmectomy (ANEURYSM-ectomy) – surgical removal of an aneurysm

aneurysmotomy (ANEURYSM-O-tomy) – surgical cutting of an aneurysm

13. VEN—vein

intravenous (*intra*-VEN-ous) – pertaining to within a vein

venule (VEN-ule) – a small vein

venoclysis (VEN-O-clysis) – irrigation of a vein, i.e., injection of fluid into a vein

14. PHLEB—vein

phlebalgia (PHLEB-algia) – painful condition (originating in a) vein

phlebophlebostomy (PHLEB-O-PHLEB-O-stomy) – making a surgical opening between one vein and another vein, i.e., making openings in two veins for the purpose of creating an artificial connection

phleboid (PHLEB-oid) – resembling a vein

15. CAPILL—hair, hairlike structure

capillaceous (CAPILL-aceous) – having hairlike structures

capillary (CAPILL-ary) – pertaining to hair or hairlike structures

The smallest blood vessels in the body are less than the thickness of a human hair in size; they are called capillaries and they connect arterioles to venules. We can think of CAPILLAR- as a base:

16. CAPILLAR—capillary

capillarectasia (CAPILLAR-ectasia) – dilation of the capillaries

capillaritis (CAPILLAR-itis) – inflammation of the capillaries

capillaropathy (CAPILLAR-O-pathy) – disease of the capillaries

17. FENESTR—window

fenestral (FENESTR-al) – pertaining to a window

In medical terminology, a windowlike opening may be called a fenestra (plural fenestrae):

FENESTR—opening, fenestra

fenestrated (FENESTR-ated) – having fenestrae

craniofenestrial (CRANI-O-FENESTR-ial) – pertaining to an opening in the skull, i.e., pertaining to incomplete formation of the bones of the fetal skull

Capillaries with small openings or pores are called fenestrated capillaries; they allow fluid transport across the capillary wall.

18. LAX—slack, loose

relaxation (*re*-LAX-ation) – process of again and again slackening, i.e., process of slackening or loosening

laxative (LAX-ative) – tending to (make) loose, i.e., making loose, usually about the bowels

19. TRACT—to pull, to draw together

contraction (*con*-TRACT-ion) – act of together drawing, i.e., act of tightening or narrowing

extractor (*ex*-TRACT-or) – thing that outward pulls, i.e., implement for pulling or drawing something out

The heart alternately contracts and relaxes in a regular rhythm. A contraction is called systole, and the period of relaxation between contractions is called diastole:

20. STOL—to send, to compress
STAL—to send, to compress

systolic (*sy*-STOL-ic) – pertaining to together sending, i.e., pertaining to contraction, pertaining to systole

diastolic (*dia*-STOL-ic) – pertaining to apart sending, i.e., pertaining to relaxation, pertaining to diastole

stalsis (STAL-sis) – process of compression, i.e., process of contraction

Note how the prefix *syn-* in systolic becomes *sy-* because the following base begins with an "s" (remember, this process is called assimilation).

21. RHYTHM—recurring motion, rhythm
-RRHYTHM—recurring motion, rhythm

anisorhythmia (ANIS-O-RHYTHM-ia) – condition of recurring motion (that is) unequal, i.e., an irregularity of the contraction and relaxation of the heart

bradydysrhythmia (BRADY-*dys*-RHYTHM-ia) – condition of abnormal rhythm (that is) slow, i.e., a slower than normal heartbeat

antiarrhythmic (*anti-a*-RRHYTHM-ic) – pertaining to against without rhythm, i.e., pertaining to counteracting abnormal heartbeat

The form -RRHYTHM- only occurs in the middle of a term, never at the beginning; it is not always used, even in the middle of a term. The term antiarrhythmic has two prefixes; remember, start with the suffix, then add the first prefix, then the second prefix, and then add in your base. In the term bradydysrhythmia, a base precedes a prefix; we use exactly the same method as we did previously—leave the base that precedes the prefix till last, treat the remaining *prefix*-BASE-suffix in the normal manner (always start with the suffix, then add the prefix, and then add in your base) and then add in the other base last.

22. POIE—to make, to form

angiopoiesis (ANGI-O-POIE-sis) – process of making (blood) vessels

leukopoietic (LEUK-O-POIE-tic) – pertaining to the process of forming white (blood cells)

galactopoiesis (GALACT-O-POIE-sis) – process of making milk

The combination of the base POIE- with the suffix -sis is a fairly common one; we can add this to our list of compound suffixes.

23. HEM—blood
HAEM—blood
HEMAT—blood
HAEMAT—blood

glycohemia (GLYC-O-HEM-ia) – condition of blood (containing) sugar

haemorrhagia (HAEM-O-rrhagia) – excessive flow of blood

hematemesis (HEMAT-emesis) – vomiting of blood

haematopoiesis (HAEMAT-O-POIE-sis) – process of making blood

You will likely come across both North American and British spellings of this base. Sometimes, the "h" of this base is dropped, especially if it occurs after a consonant:

dysaemia (*dys*-AEM-ia) – condition of abnormal blood

hyperemia (*hyper*-EM-ia) – condition of more than normal blood

The combination of the base HEM/HAEM, or the modified base EM/AEM, with the suffix -ia, meaning "condition of the blood," is a common one. We can add this to our list of compound suffixes.

24. AGOG—bringing forth, stimulating

dacryagogic (DACRY-AGOG-ic) – pertaining to stimulating tears

sialagogic (SIAL-AGOG-ic) – pertaining to stimulating saliva

hemagogic (HEM-AGOG-ic) – pertaining to bringing forth blood

You will most often see this base at the end of a term in the form -AGOGue; the ending -ue is an influence from the French language and not a proper suffix in the way that we are using them here. However, the ending -agogue, meaning "something that stimulates or promotes a flow" (hemagogue, for example), is a common one in medical terminology; we can think of it as one of the compound suffixes.

25. SANGUI—blood
SANGUIN—blood

sanguiferous (SANGUI-FER-ous) – pertaining to carrying blood

sanguinopurulent (SANGUIN-O-PUR-ulent) – full of pus and blood

exsanguination (*ex*-SANGUIN-ation) – process of outside blood, i.e., process of extensive loss of blood from the body

The major component of blood is plasma, a pale yellow colored fluid, in which cells such as erythrocytes (ERYTHR-O-cytes) and leukocytes (LEUK-O-cytes) are suspended. The plasma itself contains nutrients, proteins, hormones, clotting agents, and some waste products. We have seen the base PLAS-/PLAST- meaning "to form, to mold," and the suffix -plasm meaning "formed substance," but we can also think of PLASM-/PLASMAT- as a base:

26. PLASM—formed substance, plasma
PLASMAT—formed substance, plasma

plasmic (PLASM-ic) – pertaining to plasma

plasmatic (PLASMAT-ic) – pertaining to plasma

This base can also indicate the contents of a cell:

cytoplasmic (CYT-O-PLASM-ic) – pertaining to the formed substances (within a) cell

Blood plasma (i.e., the fluid portion of the blood) that does not contain any clotting agents is a watery substance called serum (plural sera):

27. SER—watery substance, serum

seropurulent (SER-O-PUR-ulent) – full of pus and serum

serososanguinous (SER-O-SANGUIN-ous) – pertaining to (a discharge of) blood and serum

serology (SER-O-logy) – study of sera

Sometimes, the base SER- is used about other watery substances that resemble blood serum:

serous (SER-ous) – pertaining to serum or pertaining to a watery substance (such as serum)

Serous membranes, for example, excrete substances that resemble serum and act as lubricating agents in the body.

28. DREPAN—sickle

drepanocyte (DREPAN-O-cyte) – cell that is sickle shaped

drepanocytosis (DREPAN-O-CYT-osis) – abnormal condition involving cells that are sickle shaped

A drepanocyte is a sickle- or crescent-shaped red blood cell. Drepanocytosis, or sickle cell anemia, is a hereditary blood disorder.

29. THROMB—clot

thrombocyte (THROMB-O-cyte) – cell that clots (the blood), i.e., a blood platelet

thrombocytopenia (THROMB-O-CYT-O-penia) – deficiency of the cells (responsible for blood) clotting, i.e., deficiency of blood platelets

thrombosis (THROMB-osis) – condition of a clot (formation), i.e., condition of a clot (thrombus) within a blood vessel

30. KARY—nucleus

karyolysis (KARY-O-lysis) – loosening of (the cell) nucleus, i.e., destruction of the cell nucleus

karyorrhexis (KARY-O-rrhexis) – rupture of the (cell) nucleus

megakaryocyte (MEGA-KARY-O-cyte) – cell (with a) nucleus (that is) large

Megakaryocytes are cells with large amounts of cytoplasm; sections of cytoplasm break apart and are released into the blood as cell fragments that act as thrombocytes, or blood platelets. When injury occurs, the thrombocytes clump together at the damaged site and decrease the amount of blood loss.

31. BLAST—immature cell

blastodermic (BLAST-O-DERM-ic) – pertaining to a layer of immature cells

blastoma (BLAST-oma) – mass of immature cells

You will often come across this base acting like a suffix:

erythroblast (ERYTHR-O-blast) – immature cell (that is) red, i.e., an immature red blood cell

hematoblast (HEMAT-O-blast) – immature cell of the blood

myeloblast (MYEL-O-blast) – immature cell of the bone marrow

Although it is not a true compound suffix, we will add -blast to our list.

32. EMBOL—insertion, stopper, plug

This base is really a compound of the prefix *en-*, "in," and the base BOL- meaning "to throw, to put," but the two were already put together in ancient Greek; we will treat it here as a single base. Notice how *en-* has been assimilated to *em-* before the consonant "b."

embololalia (EMBOL-O-LAL-ia) – condition of speech that inserts (meaningless words)

embolophrasia (EMBOL-O-PHRAS-ia) – condition of speech that inserts (meaningless words)

embolization (EMBOL-ization) – process of making stoppers, i.e., process of introduction of substances, usually into the circulatory system, to cause stoppages

The term embolus (plural emboli) was coined to indicate any mass of substance, whether solid, liquid, or gaseous, that could potentially block a bodily vessel, especially an artery:

EMBOL—embolus

embolemia (EMBOL-emia) – condition of the blood (carrying) emboli

embolism (EMBOL-ism) – condition of an embolus (blocking a vessel)

embolectomy (EMBOL-ectomy) – surgical removal of an embolus

33. PHAG—to eat, to ingest

dysphagia (*dys*-PHAG-ia) – condition of difficult eating, i.e., difficulty swallowing

phagocyte (PHAG-O-cyte) – cell (that) ingests, i.e., cell that ingests foreign particles

cheilophagia (CHEIL-O-PHAG-ia) – condition of eating the lip, i.e., condition of biting of the lip

coprophagy (COPR-O-PHAG-y) – condition of eating feces

The combination of the base PHAG- and the suffix -ia or -y is a common one; we can think of -phagia and -phagy as compound suffixes meaning "condition of eating." Sometimes, you will see the suffix -e added to PHAG-; as we have seen previously, the suffix -e does not have a meaning of its own, but we can treat -phage as a compound suffix meaning "thing that devours":

heterophage (HETER-O-phage) – thing that devours different (foodstuffs)

lipophage (LIP-O-phage) – thing that devours fat, i.e., a cell that ingests fat

34. SPHYGM—pulse
SPHYX—pulse

sphygmocardiograph (SPHYGM-O-CARDI-O-graph) – instrument used to record heart (beat) and pulse

anisosphygmia (ANIS-O-SPHYGM-ia) – condition of the pulse being unequal (in the arteries of two sides of the body)

sphygmoid (SPHYGM-oid) – resembling a pulse

asphyxia (*a*-SPHYX-ia) – condition of without pulse

We saw the base MAN- meaning "frenzy" and "hand" earlier, and we noted that one other meaning of this base is "thin, loose." This sense was extended to include "gas or vapor," since the atomic arrangement within them is pretty loose, and then further extended to indicate "(gas) pressure." Thus, a sphygmomanometer (SPHYGM-O-MAN-O-meter) is an "instrument used to measure the pressure of the pulse," i.e., a blood-pressure meter.

35. LYMPH—spring water, watery substance, lymph

lymphatic (LYMPH-atic) – pertaining to lymph

lymphoid (LYMPH-oid) – resembling lymph

lymphorrhagia (LYMPH-O-rrhagia) – excessive discharge of lymph (from damaged lymphatic vessels)

lymphocytopenia (LYMPH-O-CYT-O-penia) – deficiency of the cells (formed in) lymphoid tissue, i.e., deficiency of lymphocytes

Lymph is a watery fluid that seeps out of capillary walls into spaces among body tissues. It is collected and then circulated by the lymphatic vessels, and plays a major role in the body's immune system. The adenoids and tonsils (i.e., the pharyngeal, lingual, and palatine tonsils) are made up of lymphoid tissue; the thymus and the spleen are lymphoid organs:

36. SPLEN—spleen

splenomalacia (SPLEN-O-malacia) – softening of the spleen

splenoptosis (SPLEN-O-ptosis) – drooping of the spleen, i.e., downward displacement of the spleen

hypersplenia (*hyper*-SPLEN-ia) – condition of more than normal (sized) spleen

37. LIEN—spleen

lienal (LIEN-al) – pertaining to the spleen

lienometry (LIEN-O-metry) – process of measuring the spleen

lienectomy (LIEN-ectomy) – surgical removal of the spleen

You are much more likely to come across the base SPLEN- for the spleen, which has largely replaced the base LIEN-.

SOME MORE THINGS TO LEARN

Here are the compound suffixes we saw in this chapter:

1. -aemia, -emia	condition of the blood
2. -agogue	stimulating, promoting flow of
3. -blast	immature cell
4. -haemia, -hemia	condition of the blood
5. -phagia, -phagy	condition of eating
6. -phage	thing that devours
7. -poiesis	making, formation

Here are some new bases to learn. They all relate in some way to the human life span:

38. NASC—being born, birth
NAT—being born, birth

nascence (NASC-ence) – state of being born

antenatal (*ante*-NAT-al) – pertaining to before birth

perinatal (*peri*-NAT-al) – pertaining to around (the time of) birth

39. BI—(i) two, twice, double: (ii) life, living

We looked at the first meaning of BI- in a previous chapter; here, we are only concerned with its meaning "life, living."

biopsy (BI-OPS-y) – act of sight of living (tissue), i.e., examination of living tissue

biophilia (BI-O-philia) – condition of attraction for life, i.e., the instinct for self preservation

abiotic (*a*-BI-O-tic) – pertaining to the condition of without life, i.e., pertaining to the absence of life

40. PAED—child
PED—(i) child: (ii) foot

paediatrics (PAED-iatrics) – medical treatment of children
paedodontics (PAED-ODONT-ics) – study (and treatment) of teeth of children

You will likely come across both British and North American spellings of this base, but only PED- has the alternate meaning "foot," which we will come to in a later chapter. A common medical term that might be confusing is orthopedics:

orthopedics (ORTH-O-PED-ics) – science of child correcting

Originally, orthopedics dealt with the correcting of childhood deformities, but this medical specialty was extended to include the treatment of all musculo-skeletal problems in all ages of patients.

41. PUBER—coming to maturity
PUBERT—coming to maturity

impuberal (*im*-PUBER-al) – pertaining to not coming to maturity, i.e., immature
postpubertal (*post*-PUBERT-al) – pertaining to after coming to maturity, i.e., mature
puberty (PUBERT-y) – state of coming to maturity

42. GER—old age
GERONT—old age

geriatrics (GER-iatrics) – medical treatment of the aged
gerodermic (GER-O-DERM-ic) – pertaining to skin that is aged
gerontology (GERONT-O-logy) – study of old age

43. SEN—old age

senile (SEN-ile) – pertaining to old age
senopia (SEN-opia) – condition of sight (associated with) old age
senescent (SEN-escent) – becoming aged

44. PRESBY—old age

presbyacousia (PRESBY-acousia) – condition of hearing (associated with) old age
presbyopia (PRESBY-opia) – condition of sight (associated with) old age
presbycardia (PRESBY-CARD-ia) – condition of the heart (associated with) old age

45. THANAT—death

thanatology (THANAT-O-logy) – study of death and dying

thanatophoric (THANAT-O-PHOR-ic) – pertaining to carrying (toward) death, i.e., pertaining to leading to death

thanatopsy (THANAT-OPS-y) – act of sight of death, i.e., examination of a dead body

46. MORT—death, dead

premortal (*pre*-MORT-al) – pertaining to before death

mortification (MORT-I-fication) – process of becoming dead, i.e., process of death of one part of the body

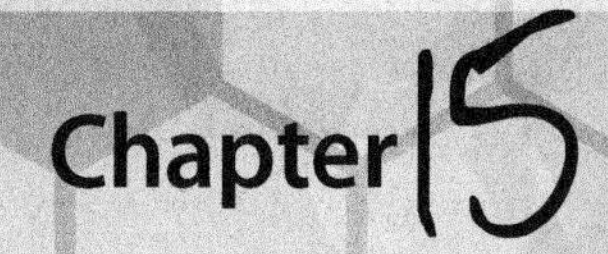

LIVER, GALLBLADDER, AND PANCREAS

SUFFIXES

There are no new suffixes to learn.

BASES

1. **HEPAT—liver**

   hepatomegaly (HEPAT-O-megaly) – enlargement of the liver

   hepatorrhexis (HEPAT-O-rrhexis) – rupture of the liver

   perihepatitis (*peri*-HEPAT-itis) – inflammation of (the covering) around the liver

2. **GER—to carry, to produce**
   GEST—to carry, to produce

   lactigerous (LACT-I-GER-ous) – pertaining to producing milk

   ingestion (*in*-GEST-ion) – act of into carrying, i.e., act of taking substances into the body

   congestive (*con*-GEST-ive) – tending to together carry, i.e., tending to accumulate a substance

   gestation (GEST-ation) – process of carrying (a fetus)

   digestion (*di*-GEST-ion) – act of apart producing, i.e., act of breaking apart food for absorption

We have already seen the base GER- meaning "old age," but context should help you figure out which base is meant. The liver, along with the gallbladder and pancreas, is an accessory organ of digestion. All three of these organs contribute to the process of digestion even though they are not physically part of it. The combination of *di-* and GEST- is so common that we can think of DIGEST- as a base:

3. **DIGEST—to break apart, to dissolve**

   indigestible (*in*-DIGEST-ible) – able to be not broken apart, i.e., not able to be broken down

   digestive (DIGEST-ive) – pertaining to breaking apart or dissolving

4. **BIL—bile**

   biliary (BIL-I-ary) – pertaining to bile

   biliptysis (BIL-I-PTY-sis) – condition of saliva (containing) bile

   bilitherapy (BIL-I-therapy) – treatment with bile (or bile salts)

   bilirubin (BIL-I-RUB-in) – substance (that is) red (in the) bile, i.e., the red bile pigment that is called bilirubin

Bile is a yellowish-brown or yellowish-green, bitter tasting fluid that is continuously produced by the liver. Along with bile acids and other fluids, bile contains the pigment bilirubin.

5. **ICTER—jaundice, icterus**

   icterogenic (ICTER-O-genic) – producing jaundice

   icterohepatitis (ICTER-O-HEPAT-itis) – inflammation of the liver (characterized by) jaundice

Jaundice, or icterus as it is sometimes called, is a yellow staining of the skin, and of the whites of the eyes. It is caused by high levels of bilirubin in the blood, and is a symptom of liver disease.

6. **CHOL—bile, gall**

   eucholia (*eu*-CHOL-ia) – condition of normal bile

   cholangiectasis (CHOL-ANGI-ectasis) – dilation of the vessel (that carries) bile, i.e., dilation of the bile duct

   cholepoiesis (CHOL-E-poiesis) – formation of bile

The pairing of the two bases CHOL- and ANGI- occurs often; together they have the meaning "bile duct": we can think of CHOLANGI- as a base:

7. **CHOLANGI—bile duct**

cholangioma (CHOLANGI-oma) – tumor of the bile duct

cholangioscopy (CHOLANGI-O-scopy) – process of examining the bile duct with an instrument

Gall is another name for bile; you will find the base CHOL- is also combined with other bases in terms that indicate the gallbladder and the gallstone. You have met the base CYST- previously, and we can think of CHOLECYST- as a new base:

8. **CHOLECYST—gallbladder**

cholecystectasia (CHOLECYST-ectasia) – dilation of the gallbladder

cholecystopathy (CHOLECYST-O-pathy) – disease of the gallbladder

cholecystopexy (CHOLECYST-O-pexy) – surgical fastening of the gallbladder (to the abdominal wall)

9. **LITH—stone, calculus**

lithogenesis (LITH-O-genesis) – production of calculi

lithodialysis (LITH-O-dialysis) – surgical dissolving of a calculus

lithotripsy (LITH-O-tripsy) – surgical crushing of a stone

cholelithic (CHOL-E-LITH-ic) – pertaining to a stone of gall, i.e., pertaining to a gallstone

cholelithotomy (CHOL-E-LITH-O-tomy) – surgical removal of a stone of gall, i.e., surgical removal of a gallstone

Look back at the base CALC- if you cannot remember where the term calculus comes from.

10. **DOCH—receptacle, duct**

sialodochoplasty (SIAL-O-DOCH-O-plasty) – surgical reshaping of the receptacle or duct for saliva, i.e., surgical reshaping or repair of the salivary duct

choledochitis (CHOL-E-DOCH-itis) – inflammation of the receptacle or duct for bile, i.e., inflammation of the bile duct

The Greek meaning of this base is receptacle; however, in medical terminology, it has also come to mean a duct that carries a substance away from a receptacle. We can think of CHOLEDOCH- as a base:

11. **CHOLEDOCH—bile duct**

choledochectomy (CHOLEDOCH-ectomy) – surgical removal of the bile duct (or part of it)

choledochostomy (CHOLEDOCH-O-stomy) – making a surgical opening into the bile duct

choledochocholedochostomy (CHOLEDOCH-O-CHOLEDOCH-O-stomy) – making a surgical opening between (one part of the) bile duct and (another part of the) bile duct, i.e., making openings in two parts of the bile duct for the purpose of creating an artificial connection

12. PANCRE—pancreas
PANCREAT—pancreas

hypopancreorrhea (*hypo*-PANCRE-O-rrhea) – flow of less than normal pancreas (secretions)

apancreatic (*a*-PANCREAT-ic) – pertaining to without a pancreas

cholangiopancreatography (CHOLANGI-O-PANCREAT-O-graphy) – process of recording the pancreas and bile duct (form and function)

pancreatolithiasis (PANCREAT-O-LITH-iasis) – abnormal condition of stones in the pancreas

The pancreas is a long, flattened gland in the abdomen that secretes digestive enzymes. Aristotle seems to have been the first to have used this word, which is actually a combination of the base PAN-, meaning "all," and a base that you have not met, KREAS- (or, CREAS-), meaning "flesh," since the pancreas was seen as an "all fleshy" gland.

13. CRIN—to secrete

crinogenic (CRIN-O-genic) – producing secretion

endocrinology (*endo*-CRIN-O-logy) – study of inside secretions, i.e., study of internal secretions of ductless glands, usually into the circulation system

exocrinologist (*exo*-CRIN-O-logist) – one who studies external secretions, i.e., one who studies external secretions made through excretory ducts

The pancreas is both an exocrine and endocrine organ in that it secretes digestive components into the pancreatic duct (exocrine function) and it secretes hormones directly into the bloodstream (endocrine function). We can think of -crine as a compound suffix made up of the base CRIN- and the suffix -e. Remember, the suffix -e does not have a meaning of its own.

14. ZYM—fermentation

zymogenic (ZYM-O-genic) – producing fermentation

zymic (ZYM-ic) – pertaining to fermentation

enzymatic (*en*-ZYM-atic) – pertaining to inward fermentation, i.e., pertaining to enzyme activity

The term enzyme was created in the 1880's to describe the vital forces involved in turning sugar into alcohol. Now, we use the term enzyme to describe a substance that accelerates chemical change. The pancreas secretes the digestive enzyme lipase.

15. ENZYM—enzyme

enzymopathy (ENZYM-O-pathy) – disease (due to) enzyme (disfunction)

enzymolysis (ENZYM-O-lysis) – loosening (of a substance) by enzymes, i.e., splitting of a substance by enzyme activity

SOME MORE THINGS TO LEARN

One of the major functions of the liver is the removal of toxic substances from the body; here are some new bases to learn that relate to things that can, in some way, be harmful to the body:

16. TOX—poison
TOXIC—poison

toxemia (TOX-emia) – condition of the blood being poisonous, i.e., condition of poisonous substances in the blood

cryptotoxic (CRYPT-O-TOX-ic) – pertaining to poisonous (properties that are) hidden

toxicodermatitis (TOXIC-O-DERMAT-itis) – inflammation of the skin (caused by) poisonous material

The original meaning of this base is "bow," and a toxophilist is someone who loves archery. However, the sense was also extended to "arrow," then "poisoned arrow" and, finally, "poison."

17. VENEN—poison

veneniferous (VENEN-I-FER-ous) – pertaining to carrying poison

venenosalivary (VENEN-O-SALIV-ary) – pertaining to saliva (that is) poisonous

venenation (VENEN-ation) – process of poisoning

18. VIR—poison
VIRUL—poisonous

virulent (VIRUL-ent) – pertaining to (being) poisonous

Originally meaning "poisonous," the term virus was later applied to any agent that caused infectious disease. It was not until the end of the 19th century that the microbes that we know today as viruses were discovered and were given this name:

VIR—virus

viropexis (VIR-O-pexis) – fixing of a virus (in a host cell)

virucopria (VIR-U-COPR-ia) – condition of the feces (containing) viruses

antiviral (*anti*-VIR-al) – pertaining to (working) against a virus

19. BOTUL—sausage

botuliform (BOTUL-I-form) – having the form of a sausage, i.e., sausage shaped

The source of an outbreak of disease in 18th century Germany was eventually traced to people having eaten bad sausages. The illness was later named botulism, after the Latin word *botulus* meaning sausage. Today, we know that this particular type of food poisoning occurs through the toxins released by a particular bacterium, and is most prevalent in improperly canned or preserved foods:

BOTUL—sausage poisoning, botulism

botulogenic (BOTUL-O-genic) – producing botulism

botulin (BOTUL-in) – substance (that causes) botulism, i.e., the botulism toxin

The botulism toxin is one of the most lethal toxins known, but it also has medicinal use in cases that benefit from its properties as a muscle relaxant. In the cosmetic industry, it goes under the name "botox," and is used to relax wrinkles.

20. ALLANT—sausage

allantoid (ALLANT-oid) – shaped like a sausage

While the term botulism now encompasses poisoning due to the botulism toxin from any source, you might also come across this base that still retains the specific sense of "sausage poisoning":

ALLANT—sausage poisoning

allantiasis (ALLANT-iasis) – abnormal condition of sausage poisoning

21. VERM—worm

vermiculus (VERM-I-culus) – small worm (or a wormlike structure)

vermiform (VERM-I-form) – like a worm, i.e., worm shaped, sometimes said of the appendix

22. HELMINTH—worm

helminthology (HELMINTH-O-logy) – study of (intestinal) worms

helminthemesis (HELMINTH-EME-sis) – condition of vomiting worms

helminthophobia (HELMINTH-O-phobia) – abnormal fear of worms

23. ACAR—mite, tick

acarodermatitis (ACAR-O-DERMAT-itis) – inflammation of the skin (caused by) mites

acariasis (ACAR-iasis) – abnormal condition (caused by) mites

acarology (ACAR-O-logy) – study of mites and ticks (and the diseases they transmit)

24. MYI—fly

myiasis (MYI-A-sis) – condition (caused by) fly (larvae)

Be careful not to confuse this base with MY- meaning muscle; myiasis is probably the only term in medical terminology where you will come across the base MYI-.

25. BACTERI—staff, cane, rod

Though bacteria had first been observed in the 17th century, it was not until the 19th century that they got their present name; the name bacteria (singular bacterium) reflects the fact that most of the earliest discoveries were rod-shaped microorganisms:

BACTERI—bacterium

bactericholia (BACTERI-CHOL-ia) – condition of the bile (containing) bacteria

antibacterial (*anti*-BACTERI-al) – pertaining to (working) against bacteria

bacterioclasis (BACTERI-O-clasis) – breakage of bacteria, i.e., fragmentation of bacteria

26. BACILL—rod, stick

bacillar (BACILL-ar) – pertaining to rod(-shaped)

bacilliform (BACILL-I-form) – having the form of a rod, i.e., rod shaped

You will come across this base most often in terms related to bacillus (plural bacilli), the name given to a rod-shaped bacterium:

BACILL—rod-shaped bacterium, bacillus

bacillosis (BACILL-osis) – abnormal condition (caused by) bacilli

bacillemia (BACILL-emia) – condition of the blood (caused by the presence) of bacilli

necrobacillosis (NECR-O-BACILL-osis) – abnormal condition (caused by) bacilli (that leads to tissue) death

There is another base that means "rod"; it is not directly related to the conditions we are talking about here but it we will look at it here anyway:

27. RHABD—rod, stick

rhabdoid (RHABD-oid) – shaped like a rod

rhabdophobia (RHABD-O-phobia) – abnormal fear of (being beaten by a) stick

rhabdomyoma (RHABD-O-MY-oma) – a tumor in muscle (that has) rod (shaped cells), i.e., a tumor in skeletal muscle

rhabdomyolysis (RHABD-O-MY-O-lysis) – loosening of muscles (that have) rod (shaped cells), i.e., destruction of skeletal muscle

Skeletal muscles are generally composed of long, rod-shaped cells; the base RHABD-, often combined with the base MY-, indicates skeletal muscle.

28. COCC—seed, berry

The original meaning of this base is seed or berry; however, in medical terminology, this has been extended to "berry shaped" and is often applied to "berry-shaped (i.e., round) bacteria":

COCC—berry shaped, coccus (a berry-shaped bacterium, plural cocci)

coccal (COCC-al) – pertaining to a coccus

coccoid (COCC-oid) – shaped like a coccus

pyococcal (PY-O-COCC-al) – pertaining to a coccus (that forms) pus

meningococcal (MENING-O-COCC-al) – pertaining to a coccus (that attacks the) meninges

Generally, a coccus is a bacterium that is round or spheroidal; a coccobacillus has a shape in-between a coccus and a bacillus, that is, a short rod with rounded ends. The term coccus can also be used about other round or spherical organisms:

cryptococcosis (CRYPT-O-COCC-osis) – abnormal condition (caused by a) berry-shaped (yeast that is) hidden (within a capsule)

Cryptococcus is a yeast (a member of the fungus family) with a round shape and it is surrounded by an enveloping capsule.

coccidium (COCC-idium) – small berry-shaped (protozoan)

Coccidia (singular coccidium) are protozoa (single-celled organisms) with a round shape; they live as parasites in the intestines of many animals and can cause a variety of diseases termed coccidiosis. Some species of coccidia are transferrable to humans. Be careful not to confuse COCC- with the base COCCY- meaning "cuckoo" or, more frequently, "coccyx, tail bone."

29. STREP—curved, twisted, linked
STREPT—curved, twisted, linked

phlebostrepsis (PHLEB-O-STREP-sis) – condition of twisted vein, i.e., twisting a cut end of a vein to prevent hemorrhage

This base is generally used about organisms that have a curved or twisted shape. Certain types of cocci (berry-shaped bacteria) grow in chains that can take on curved or twisted formations; they are termed streptococci:

streptococcosis (STREPT-O-COCC-osis) – abnormal condition (due to) cocci that are twisted, i.e., abnormal condition due to streptococci

Sometimes, you will find that the base STREPT- is used on its own to denote the streptococci bacteria:

STREPT—streptococcus

streptodermatitis (STREPT-O-DERMAT-itis) – inflammation of the skin due to streptococci

Earlier we saw the base STAPHYL- meaning "bunch of grapes" (extended to denote the uvula). While streptococci are bacteria that form curved chains, staphylococci grow in clumps that resemble bunches of grapes.

30. PHYT—plant

phytodermatitis (PHYT-O-DERMAT-itis) – inflammation of the skin (due to contact with) plants

phytophagous (PHYT-O-PHAG-ous) – pertaining to eating plants, i.e., vegetarian

This base is related to the base PHY-, "to grow," that we saw earlier. Sometimes, you will see the suffix -e added to PHYT-; as we have seen previously, the suffix -e does not have a meaning of its own, but we can treat -phyte as a compound suffix meaning "plant" or "growth":

coprophyte (COPR-O-phyte) – plant (that lives on) dung

osteophyte (OSTE-O-phyte) – growth of bone, i.e., a bony outgrowth

31. FUNG—mushroom, fungus

fungal (FUNG-al) – pertaining to a fungus

fungemia (FUNG-emia) – condition of the blood (carrying) fungi

fungitoxic (FUNG-I-TOX-ic) – pertaining to poisonous to fungus (growth)

Note that fungitoxic denotes something that is poisonous to fungi, not a fungus that is poisonous to humans.

32. MYC—fungus
MYCET—fungus

mycotoxicosis (MYC-O-TOXIC-osis) – condition of poisoning (due to) fungi

oculomycosis (OCUL-O-MYC-osis) – condition of fungal (infection) of the eye

mycetophagous (MYCET-O-PHAG-ous) – pertaining to eating fungi

33. SPOR—seed, spore

sporogenesis (SPOR-O-genesis) – production of spores

trichosporosis (TRICH–O-SPOR-osis) – condition of (fungal) spore (infection) of the hair

34. SEP—to rot, to putrefy

antisepsis (*anti*-SEP-sis) – process of against putrefying, i.e., preventing infection by inhibiting infecting elements

septic (SEP-tic) – pertaining to the process of putrefaction, i.e., pertaining to toxins being produced

septicemia (SEP-tic-emia) – condition of the blood pertaining to process of putrefaction, i.e., toxins circulating in the bloodstream

35. CID—to cut, to kill
CIS—to cut, to kill

excision (*ex*-CIS-ion) – act of out cutting, i.e., cutting out, surgical removal

bacteriocidal (BACTERI-O-CID-al) – pertaining to killing bacteria

The two meanings of this base are connected since, in earlier times, one way to kill someone was to cut them down with a sword. You will probably come across this base most often as the compound suffix -cide, meaning "killing" or "substance that kills":

fungicide (FUNG-I-cide) – substance that kills fungi

vermicide (VERM-I-cide) – substance that kills (intestinal) worms

sporicide (SPOR-I-cide) – substance that kills spores

36. FUG—to flee from, to put to flight

vermifugal (VERM-I-FUG-al) – pertaining to putting to flight (intestinal) worms, i.e., pertaining to expelling intestinal worms

You will probably come across this base most often as the compound suffix -fuge, meaning "substance that expels" or "substance that drives away":

lactifuge (LACT-I-fuge) – substance that drives away milk, i.e., substance that lessens milk secretion

vermifuge (VERM-I-fuge) – substance that expels (intestinal) worms

We saw the base STA- previously, meaning "to stand," and the related compound suffixes -stasia, -stasis, and -stasy meaning "stoppage, stagnation"; the ending -stat is not a true compound suffix in the way we have described them but it occurs quite often as an ending meaning "agent that inhibits, agent that retards":

bacteriostat (BACTERI-O-stat) – agent that inhibits bacteria, i.e., agent that retards bacterial growth

mycostat (MYC-O-stat) – agent that inhibits fungi, i.e., agent that retards fungal growth

fungistat (FUNG-I-stat) – agent that inhibits fungi, i.e., agent that retards fungal growth

Therefore, we will add it to our list of new compound suffixes:

1. -cide	killing, substance that kills
2. -crine	thing that secretes
3. -fuge	substance that expels, substance that drives away
4. -phyte	plant, growth
5. -stat	agent that inhibits, agent that retards

We have covered another five chapters since the last review, so this seems like a good place for another summary of some of the topics we have covered.

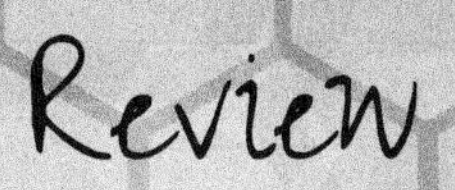

CHAPTERS 11–15

PREFIXES

We did not add any new prefixes to our list.

SUFFIXES

Let us add the new suffixes we have learned in the previous five chapters to our lists.

ADJECTIVE-FORMING SUFFIXES

All of these suffixes form an adjective when added to a base:

1. -able, -abil-	able to be
2. -ac	pertaining to
3. -aceous	pertaining to, belonging to, having
4. -acious	tending to, inclined to
5. -ad	toward
6. -al, -eal, -ial	pertaining to
7. -alis, -aris	pertaining to
8. -an	pertaining to
9. -ant	pertaining to

10. -ar	pertaining to, having the character of
11. -ary	pertaining to
12. -ate	pertaining to, having, having the shape, to (...)
13. -ated	composed of, having
14. -atic	pertaining to
15. -ative	pertaining to, tending to
16. -atory	pertaining to
17. -ent	pertaining to
18. -escent	beginning to be, becoming
19. -etic	pertaining to
20. -fic	causing, making
21. -form	having the form of, like
22. -ian	pertaining to
23. -iatic	pertaining to a state, pertaining to a process
24. -ible, -ibil-	able to be
25. -ic	pertaining to
26. -ical	pertaining to
27. -id	pertaining to, having
28. -ile	pertaining to, able to be
29. -ine	pertaining to
30. -ior	pertaining to
31. -ious	pertaining to
32. -ive	pertaining to, tending to
33. -oid	resembling, shaped, like, shaped like
34. -ory	having the function of
35. -ose	full of, having the quality of

36. -ous	pertaining to, like, full of, having
37. -tic	pertaining to
38. -ual	pertaining to
39. -ulent	full of

Remember, the suffix -ate can also be a verb-forming suffix meaning "to do, to cause."

NOUN-FORMING SUFFIXES

All of these suffixes form a noun when added to a base:

40. -ance, -ancy	state of
41. -ase	enzyme (chemistry)
42. -ation	process
43. -ator	person who (does…), thing that (does…)
44. -ature	system composed of
45. -duct	duct, channel, tube
46. -ema	condition
47. -ence	state of
48. -er	person who (does…), thing that (does…)
49. -esis	condition, abnormal condition, process
50. -ety	condition, state, quality
51. -fication	process of producing, process of becoming, process of making
52. -gen	that which produces
53. -gram	record
54. -graph	instrument used to record
55. -ia	state of, condition of, quality of, act of

56. -iasis	state of, process of, abnormal condition
57. -ician	specialist
58. -ics, -tics	art of, science of, study of
59. -in	substance
60. -ion	action, condition, act of
61. -ism	condition of
62. -ist	person who (does…), specialist
63. -itis	inflammation
64. -ity	condition, state, quality
65. -ization	process of making
66. -ment	action of, product of
67. -meter	instrument used to measure
68. -ol	alcohol (chemistry)
69. -oma	tumor, mass
70. -one	ketone (chemistry)
71. -or	person who (does…), thing that (does…)
72. -orium	place for
73. -ose	sugar (chemistry)
74. -osis	process of, condition of, abnormal condition of
75. -plasm	formed substance, growth
76. -scope	instrument used to examine
77. -sia, -sis	process of, condition of, act of
78. -um	structure, substance
79. -ure	result of, act of
80. -y	state of, condition of, quality of, act of

These diminutive forming suffixes also make nouns when added to a base:

81. -cle	small
82. -culus, -cula, -culum	small
83. -ellus, -ella, -ellum	small
84. -idium	small
85. -il	small
86. -illus, -illa, -illum	small
87. -ium	small
88. -ole	small
89. -ule	small
90. -ulus, -ula, -ulum	small
91. -uncle	small
92. -unculus	small

VERB-FORMING SUFFIXES

All of these suffixes form a verb when added to a base:

93. -ate	pertaining to, having, having the shape, to (...)
94. -esce	to begin, to become
95. -fy	to produce, to become, to make
96. -ize	to make, to affect
97. -verse	to turn, to travel turned

Remember, the suffix -ate can also be an adjective-forming suffix meaning "pertaining to, having."

COMPOUND SUFFIXES

Some base-suffix pairs occur together so regularly that they are often treated as one suffix, and we have used the term compound suffix to describe them. Here are the compound suffixes that we have seen, but bear in mind that this is just a list created for this present task in medical terminology. In a different discipline, the list of compound suffixes would be quite different.

Remember, it is helpful to memorize all the compound suffixes because they occur so regularly, but you can also always build them up from their individual base and suffix parts.

Most of the compound suffixes we have made are nouns. Here are the ones that relate to the senses and the mind:

1. -acousia	condition of hearing
2. -blepsia	condition of sight
3. -esthesia	condition of sensation
4. -geusia	condition of sense of taste
5. -mania	condition of madness, compulsion, obsession
6. -mnesia	condition of memory, memory
7. -opia	condition of sight
8. -opsia	condition of sight
9. -osmia	condition of sense of smell
10. -philia	condition of attraction, abnormal craving for
11. -phobia	condition of fear, abnormal fear of

Here are the ones that relate to medical procedures and treatment:

12. -agogue	stimulating, promoting flow of
13. -centesis	surgical puncturing, puncturing
14. -cide	killing, substance that kills
15. -clasia, -clasis	surgical fracture, breaking, rupture

16. -cleisis	surgical closure, closure
17. -clysis	therapeutic infusion of liquid, irrigation
18. -desis	surgical fusion, binding
19. -dialysis	surgical dissolving, surgical separation, filtration
20 -ectomy	surgical removal, removal
21. -fuge	substance that expels, substance that drives away
22. -iatrics, -iatry	medical treatment
23. -lysis	surgical dissolving, surgical separation, loosening
24. -pexis, -pexy	surgical fastening, fixing
25. -plasia, -plasty	surgical reshaping, formation
26. -stat	agent that inhibits, agent that retards
27. -stomy	making a surgical opening, making an opening
28. -therapia, -therapy	treatment
29. -tripsy	surgical crushing, crushing
30. -tomy	surgical cutting, cutting

Here are the ones that express some physical condition:

31. -agra	pain, painful seizure
32. -algesia	sensation of pain
33. -algia	painful condition
34. -asthenia	weakness
35. -atrophia, -atrophy	wasting
36. -dactylia, -dactyly	condition of the fingers or toes
37. -dystrophia, -dystrophy	weakness
38. -ectasia, -ectasis	expansion, widening, dilation
39. -ectopia, -ectopy	displacement

40. -emesia, -emesis	vomiting
41. -emphraxis	obstruction
42. -(h)aemia, -(h)emia	condition of the blood
43. -lepsis, -lepsy	seizure
44. -malacia	softening
45. -megaly	enlargement
46. -nosia	disease
47. -odynia	painful condition
48. -(o)edema	swelling
49. -pathia, -pathy	disease, treatment of disease
50. -penia	deficiency
51. -phthisis	wasting
52. -plegia	paralysis
53. -plexia, -plexy	seizure
54. -ptosia, -ptosis	drooping, prolapse
55. -schisis	fissure
56. -stasia, -stasis, -stasy	stoppage, stagnation
57. -stenosis	narrowing, contraction
58. -syndactylia, -syndactyly	condition of fused fingers or toes

The -rrh compounds are not true compound suffixes in the way we have described them, but they do occur quite often, so it is good to be aware of them:

59. -rrhage	excessive flow, excessive discharge
60. -rrhagia	excessive flow, excessive discharge
61. -rrhaphy	surgical suture
62. -rrhea	flow, discharge
63. -rrhexis	rupture

Here are the remaining compound suffixes that form nouns:

64. -blast	immature cell
65. -crine	thing that secretes
66. -cyte	cell
67. -genesis	production
68. -graphy	process of recording
69. -gravida	woman who is, or has been, pregnant
70. -logist	one who studies
71. -logy	study of
72. -metry	process of measuring
73. -para	woman who has given birth
74. -phage	thing that devours
75. -phagia, -phagy	condition of eating
76. -phyte	plant, growth
77. -pnea	breathing, respiration
78. -poiesis	making, formation
79. -scopy	process of examining with an instrument
80. -tome	instrument used to cut

These compound suffixes form adjectives:

81. -genic	producing, produced
82. -genous	producing, produced
83. -verse	to turn, to travel, turned

BUILDING UP MEDICAL DEFINITIONS

We have now seen this term:

> acrocephalopolysyndactyly (ACR-O-CEPHAL-O-POLY-*syn*-DACTYL-y) – condition of together fingers or toes—many of them, and a head that is (like) the highest point, i.e., condition involving several fused fingers or toes and a head that is peak shaped

It has the form (excluding combining vowels) BASE-BASE-BASE-*prefix*-BASE-suffix. We approached it as a regular *prefix*-BASE-suffix type and then added in the other bases going from right to left. We were able to use and to join in one of the bases, but we had to use some common sense to help us add in the other bases.

We have also seen terms involving two bases and a prefix where the prefix does not modify the ultimate base. In both atelencephalia and ataxiaphasia, the prefix *a*- modifies the base closest to it. You will find that this is often the case with the prefix *a*-.

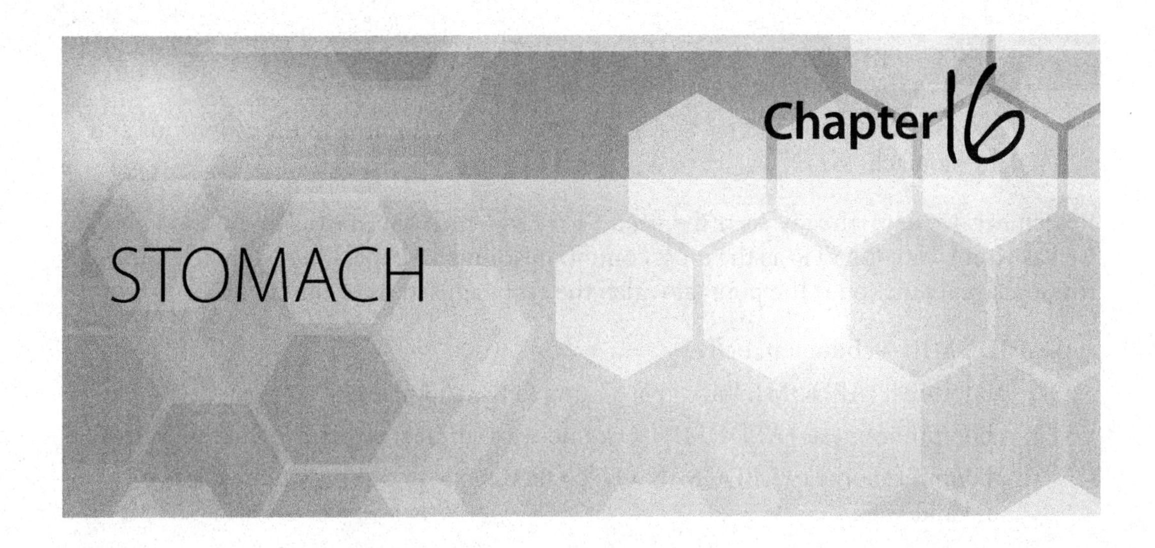

The term stomach derives from the little used base STOMACH-, originally meaning "gullet" but later extended to the organ we know by this name today. You may come across the terms stomachic (STOMACH-ic) and stomachal (STOMACH-al) meaning "pertaining to the stomach," but probably not much else. In medical terminology, stomach is a precise term, but in everyday language it is often quite vague, variously indicating an area somewhere between chest and pelvis. Medically, the stomach is the organ of digestion located between the esophagus and the small intestine.

BASES

1. **ESOPHAG—gullet, esophagus**
   OESOPHAG—gullet, esophagus

    esophageal (ESOPHAG-eal) – pertaining to the esophagus

    esophagostenosis (ESOPHAG-O-stenosis) – narrowing of the esophagus

    oesophagomalacia (OESOPHAG-O-malacia) – softening of the esophagus (walls)

You may still come across the British spelling OESOPHAG- (and oesophagus), but the North American spelling has largely been adopted. This base is related to PHAG-, "to eat, to ingest," that we saw previously.

2. **GASTR—stomach**

    gastrodynia (GASTR-odynia) – painful condition of the stomach

    gastrohepatic (GASTR-O-HEPAT-ic) – pertaining to the liver and stomach cholecystogastrostomy (CHOLECYST-O-GASTR-O-stomy) – making a surgical opening (between) the stomach and the gallbladder

gastroesophageal (GASTR-O-ESOPHAG-eal) – pertaining to the esophagus and the stomach

Remember, we have already seen the base VENTR- which can mean "belly, abdomen," as well as "front," but GASTR- is the most commonly found base meaning "stomach." The gastroesophageal junction is the point at which the esophagus joins to the stomach.

3. ABDOMIN—abdomen, belly

abdominal (ABDOMIN-al) – pertaining to the abdomen

abdominocentesis (ABDOMIN-O-centesis) – surgical puncturing of the abdomen

abdominothoracic (ABDOMIN-O-THORAC-ic) – pertaining to the chest and abdomen

Like the term stomach in everyday language, the abdomen can also be a tricky area to pin down; it most often refers to an area between the chest and pelvis (not including the vertebral region), although sometimes it is extended to include the pelvis as well.

4. CEL—abdomen, belly, abdominal cavity
CELI—abdomen, belly, abdominal cavity
COEL—abdomen, belly, abdominal cavity
COELI—abdomen, belly, abdominal cavity

celitis (CEL-itis) – inflammation of the abdomen

celiomyalgia (CELI-O-MY-algia) – painful condition of the muscles of the abdomen

coeliac (COEL-I-ac) – pertaining to the abdomen or abdominal cavity

coelioscopy (COELI-O-scopy) – process of examining the abdomen with an instrument

Again, the North American spellings (CEL- and CELI-) have largely replaced the British forms (COEL- and COELI-). You may also come across this base at the end of a term, where it always has the meaning "cavity":

-COEL cavity

-COELE cavity

hemocoel (HEM-O-COEL) – cavity (containing) blood

blastocoele (BLAST-O-COELE) – cavity in immature cells, i.e., the first cavity in an early stage embryo

Although it is not a true compound suffix, we will add -coel/-coele to our list. You may also come across -cele as an alternative spelling, as in blastocele; in most cases, however, -cele has a different meaning:

CELE– hernia, protrusion, swelling

arthrocele (ARTHR-O-CELE) – swelling of a joint

encephalocele (ENCEPHAL-O-CELE) – hernia of the brain

meningomyelocele (MENING-O-MYEL-O-CELE) – protrusion of the spinal cord and the spinal meninges (through the spinal column)

Again, although it is not a true compound suffix, we will add -cele to our list.

5. **UMBILIC—navel, belly button, umbilicus**

   umbilical (UMBILIC-al) – pertaining to the navel

   umbilicate (UMBILIC-ate) – having the shape of a navel

The most common medical term for the navel or belly button is the umbilicus. In compound terms, however, you are more likely to see the base OMPHAL-:

6. **OMPHAL—navel, umbilicus, umbilical cord**

   omphalocele (OMPHAL-O-cele) – hernia of the navel

   omphalotripsy (OMPHAL-O-tripsy) – surgical crushing of the umbilical cord

   omphalophlebitis (OMPHAL-O-PHLEB-itis) – inflammation of the veins of the umbilicus

Occasionally, you may come across the term omphalos instead of umbilicus for the navel.

7. **LAPAR—abdomen, loin**

   laparocele (LAPAR-O-cele) – hernia of the abdomen

   laparomyositis (LAPAR-O-MYOS-itis) – inflammation of the muscles of the abdomen

   laparotomy (LAPAR-O-tomy) – surgical cutting of the abdomen or loin

Once again, the exact area that this base refers to can be difficult to pin down. Originally meaning the soft parts between the ribs and the hips, it can now refer to the abdomen, to the loin (another indeterminate area), or to parts in-between.

8. **PORT—gate, point of entry**

portal (PORT-al) – pertaining to a gate

In medical terminology, a porta (plural portae) is a point of entry or exit in the body or organs. The portal vein conducts blood from the intestines to the liver. In compound medical terms, the base PORT- generally denotes the portal vein:

PORT—portal vein

portography (PORT-O-graphy) – process of recording (the structure and functioning of) the portal vein

portobilioarterial (PORT-O-BIL-I-O-ARTER-ial) – pertaining to the (hepatic) artery, bile (ducts) and the portal vein

Note how portobilioarterial has two combining vowels between the bases BIL- and ARTER-. There is another base, PYL-, which also means "gate," and it too is used to denote the portal vein:

9. **PYL—gate, portal vein**

pylethrombosis (PYL-E-THROMB-osis) – condition of a clot in the portal vein

pylemphraxis (PYL-emphraxis) – obstruction of the portal vein

The base PYLOR-, "gatekeeper," is related to this base:

10. **PYLOR—gatekeeper**

In medical terminology, a pylorus is a muscular device that can open and close the opening of an organ; it acts like a gatekeeper. In the stomach, a pylorus controls the outlet of material from the stomach:

PYLOR—pylorus

pyloric (PYLOR-ic) – pertaining to the pylorus

pyloroptosis (PYLOR-O-ptosis) – prolapse of the pylorus

pylorectomy (PYLOR-ectomy) – surgical removal of the pylorus

The muscle that allows the pylorus to open and close is known as a sphincter muscle, derived from a base meaning "band," i.e., something that binds tightly or constricts. Most sphincter muscles occur in the digestive system:

11. **SPHINCTER—band, sphincter, sphincter muscle**

sphincteral (SPHINCTER-al) – pertaining to a sphincter

sphincterotome (SPHINCTER-O-tome) – instrument used to cut a sphincter

blepharosphincterectomy (BLEPHAR-O-SPHINCTER-ectomy) – surgical removal of (part of) the sphincter muscle of the eyelid

The stomach is divided into four regions, the cardia, fundus, body, and pylorus. We came across the term cardia previously, when we looked at the bases CARD- and CARDI-, and we have just met the term pylorus. The fundus is the uppermost part of the stomach, responsible for storing undigested food and accumulated gas. In everyday speech, the base FUND- has the meaning "depth" or "bottom," as in fundamental and profundity, but in medical terminology it almost always has the meaning "fundus." A fundus is generally the bottom or lowest part of an organ, but it can also indicate the part most remote from the opening, as is the case in the stomach:

12. FUND—fundus

fundic (FUND-ic) – pertaining to a fundus

fundiform (FUND-I-form) – having the form of a fundus

The lining of the stomach is gathered into thick, wrinklelike folds called rugae (singular ruga). They allow the stomach to expand when it becomes filled with food by unfolding:

13. RUG—wrinkle, fold

rugose (RUG-ose) – full of wrinkles

rugate (RUG-ate) – having wrinkles

corrugator (*cor*-RUG-ator) – thing that together wrinkles, i.e., a muscle that wrinkles the skin

Note how the prefix *con*- has been assimilated to *cor*- in the term corrugator.

14. CHY—to pour

You may never come across this base, meaning "to pour," in this form, but it does give us two related bases, CHYL- and CHYM-, both of which can mean "juice" or "fluid" (literally, "something that can be poured"). More specifically, these bases refer to chyle and chyme, two fluids that are associated with the process of digestion. Chyle is a milky fluid formed in the small intestine during digestion, while chyme is the semi-fluid mass of partially digested food, saliva, and gastric juices that passes from the stomach to the small intestine:

CHYL—juice, fluid, chyle
CHYM—juice, fluid, chyme

chyliferous (CHYL-I-FER-ous) – pertaining to carrying chyle

chylemia (CHYL-emia) – condition of the blood (containing) chyle

chymorrhea (CHYM-O-rrhea) – flow of chyme
chymopoiesis (CHYM-O-poiesis) – formation of chyme

Here are a couple of bases that refer to internal organs in general, including the stomach:

15. VISCER—internal organ, viscera

visceral (VISCER-al) – pertaining to the viscera
eviscerate (*e*-VISCER-ate) – to make without internal organs, i.e., to remove the internal organs
visceromegaly (VISCER-O-megaly) – enlargement of an internal organ

The term viscus (plural viscera) may be used about any of the internal organs of the thoracic and abdominopelvic cavities (i.e., within the chest, abdomen, or pelvis).

16. SPLANCHN—internal organ, viscera

splanchnic (SPLANCHN-ic) – pertaining to the viscera
splanchnocele (SPLANCHN-O-cele) – hernia of an internal organ
splanchnectopia (SPLANCHN-ectopia) – displacement of an internal organ

The following bases refer generally to food and drink, and to digestion:

17. PEPS—digestion
PEPT—digestion

pepsin (PEPS-in) – substance (related to) digestion
dyspepsia (*dys*-PEPS-ia) – condition of painful digestion
bradypepsia (BRADY-PEPS-ia) – condition of digestion that is slow
peptic (PEPT-ic) – pertaining to digestion

Pepsin is an enzyme released by the stomach that is involved in the digestion of proteins.

18. ALIMENT—food, nourishment, nutrition

alimentary (ALIMENT-ary) – pertaining to nourishment
hypoalimentation (*hypo*-ALIMENT-ation) – process of less than normal nourishment, i.e., inadequate nourishment
alimentotherapy (ALIMENT-O-therapy) – treatment (of disease) by nourishment, i.e., treatment by regulation of diet

The digestive tract, i.e., the entire passageway along which food passes, both above and below the stomach, is also known as the alimentary canal.

19. NUTRI—to nourish, nourishment
NUTRIT—to nourish, nourishment

nutrient (NUTRI-ent) – pertaining to nourishment

nutritive (NUTRIT-ive) – tending to nourish, pertaining to nourishment

malnutrition (*mal*-NUTRIT-ion) – condition of inadequate nourishment

20. SIT—food, grain

sitotoxism (SIT-O-TOX-ism) – condition of poisoning through (spoiled) grain or food

apositia (*apo*-SIT-ia) – condition of away from food, i.e., lack of appetite

sitotropic (SIT-O-TROP-ic) – pertaining to turning towards, or away from, food

21. CIB—food, meal

cibophobia (CIB-O-phobia) – abnormal fear of food, i.e., a loathing for food

postcibal (*post*-CIB-al) – pertaining to after a meal

22. ORECT—appetite
OREX—appetite

anorexia (*an*-OREX-ia) – condition of without appetite

anorectic (*an*-ORECT-ic) – pertaining to without appetite

hyperorexia (*hyper*-OREX-ia) – condition of more than normal appetite

The eating disorder that we hear a lot about is more properly called anorexia nervosa.

23. LIM—hunger

limosis (LIM-osis) – abnormal condition of hunger

limophthisis (LIM-O-phthisis) – wasting through hunger, i.e., emaciation caused by insufficient food

Another name for the eating disorder hyperorexia is boulimia nervosa; the term boulimia (or bulimia) includes the base LIM- and the base BOU- that means "ox," so BOU-LIM-ia is, literally, a "condition of hunger like an ox." You will not likely come across the base BOU- in any other medical terminology.

24. DIPS—thirst

dipsesis (DIPS-esis) – abnormal condition of thirst

adipsia (*a*-DIPS-ia) – condition of without thirst

polydipsia (POLY-DIPS-ia) – condition of thirst–much (of it), i.e., excessive thirst

The meaning of this base is sometimes extended to mean "drinking":

DIPS—drinking

dipsomania (DIPS-O-mania) – compulsion for drinking (alcohol to excess)

25. PYR—fire, burning

pyrosis (PYR-osis) – condition of burning, i.e., the condition generally known as heartburn

antipyrotic (*anti*-PYR-O-tic) – pertaining to against burning, i.e., acting to alleviate burns

pyromania (PYR-O-mania) – compulsion to set fires

Pyrosis, or heartburn, is a burning sensation in the esophagus caused by a reflux (literally, a "flowing back") of stomach acid.

26. GURGIT—to flood, to gorge

ingurgitation (*in*-GURGIT-ation) - process of in gorging, i.e., process of taking in food or drink greedily

regurgitation (*re*-GURGIT-ation) – process of backward flooding, i.e., reflux of food and/or stomach acid into the mouth, or a backward flow of blood through faulty heart valves

SOME MORE THINGS TO LEARN

We saw the base PYR- above meaning "fire, burning": closely related are the bases PYRET- and PYREX-:

27. PYRET—fever
PYREX—fever

antipyretic (*anti*-PYRET-ic) – pertaining to (working) against fever, i.e., reducing fever

pyrexia (PYREX-ia) – condition of fever

hyperpyrexial (*hyper*-PYREX-ial) – pertaining to more than normal fever, i.e., pertaining to an extremely high fever

Here is another base that means fever:

28. FEBR—fever

afebrile (*a*-FEBR-ile) – pertaining to without a fever
febrifuge (FEBR-I-fuge) – substance that drives away fever
febriferous (FEBR-I-FER-ous) – pertaining to producing fever

We have seen the combination of FER- and -ous quite a few times now, meaning "pertaining to bearing, carrying or producing"; we can add it to our list of compound suffixes. A similar way of saying "something that causes or makes something" uses the following base:

29. FAC—to make, to cause

febrifacient (FEBR-I-FAC-I-ent) – pertaining to causing fever

FAC- is related to the suffix -fic that we have already seen. We can add -facient, "making, causing," to our list of compound suffixes.

30. PHLOG—inflamed, inflammation
PHLOGIST—inflamed, inflammation

phlogocyte (PHLOG-O-cyte) – cell in inflamed (tissue)
phlogogenic (PHLOG-O-genic) – producing inflammation
antiphlogistic (*anti*-PHLOGIST-ic) – pertaining to (working) against inflammation

Here are some bases related to temperature and heat:

31. THERM- heat

thermoesthesia (THERM-O-esthesia) – condition of sensation to heat
thermotherapy (THERM-O-therapy) – treatment with heat
hypothermia (*hypo*-THERM-ia) – condition of less than normal (body) heat

32. CAL—heat
CALOR—heat

calefacient (CAL-E-facient) – making heat
calorific (CALOR-I-fic) – causing heat
calorimeter (CALOR-I-meter) – instrument used to measure heat

33. CAUM—heat, burning
CAUS—heat, burning
CAUST—heat, burning

caumesthesia (CAUM-esthesia) – condition of sensation to heat

causalgia (CAUS-algia) – painful condition of burning (sensation)

caustic (CAUST-ic) – pertaining to burning, i.e., pertaining to an effect that resembles burning

The term caumesthesia is generally used about an individual having a sensation of heat even when the temperature is low. The base CAUTER- is related to these forms; coming from the Greek term for a branding iron, it gives us the term cautery (CAUTER-y), which can mean either the instrument used to apply heat to a tissue, or the actual use of the instrument:

34. CAUTER—cautery

cauterization (CAUTER-ization) – process of making (use of) the cautery, i.e., the act of cauterizing

cauterant (CAUTER-ant) – pertaining to cautery

Cauterization can be used to seal wounds and blood vessels, and to destroy diseased or unnatural tissue. It often employs direct heat to achieve this, but cold, electric current, high frequency light, and certain chemicals may also be used.

35. CRY—icy cold
CRYM—icy cold

crymophilic (CRYM-O-PHIL-ic) – pertaining to loving icy cold (temperatures)

crymodynia (CRYM-odynia) – painful condition (due to) icy cold (temperature)

cryothalamectomy (CRY-O-THALAM-ectomy) – removal of the thalamus by icy cold (temperature)

cryolysis (CRY-O-lysis) – loosening (by) icy cold, i.e., destruction by cold

cryogenic (CRY-O-genic) – producing icy cold

A cryogen is capable of producing icy cold temperatures, and the science of cryogenics is concerned with the production of, and effects of, very low temperatures. In cryosurgery, a cryogen (very often liquid nitrogen) is used to create temperatures that are low enough to destroy diseased or unwanted tissues. You may occasionally see these two bases with a "k" replacing the letter "c" (KRY-, KRYM-).

36. PSYCHR—cold

psychroalgia (PSYCHR-O-algia) – painful condition (due to) cold
psychrophobia (PSYCHR-O-phobia) – abnormal fear of the cold

Be careful not to confuse this base with PSYCH-.

Finally, here are the new compound suffixes we saw in this chapter:

1. -cele	hernia, protrusion, swelling
2. -coel, -coele	cavity
3. -facient	making, causing
4. -ferous	bearing, carrying, producing

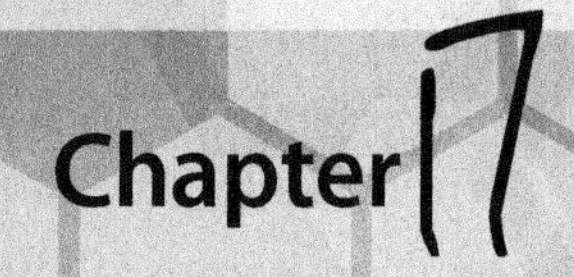

ABDOMEN AND THE DIGESTIVE ORGANS

BASES

1. **ENTER—intestine**

   enteric (ENTER-ic) – pertaining to the intestine

   enteroenterostomy (ENTER-O-ENTER-O-stomy) – making a surgical opening between (one part of) the intestine and (another part of) the intestine

   enterostenosis (ENTER-O-stenosis) – narrowing of the intestine

   parenteral (*par*-ENTER-al) – pertaining to beside the intestines

2. **INTESTIN—intestine**

   intestinal (INTESTIN-al) – pertaining to the intestine

   gastrointestinal (GASTR-O-INTESTIN-al) – pertaining to the intestine and stomach

This base only rarely appears in compound terms. Both ENTER- and INTESTIN- often indicate the small intestine specifically, but this is not always the case; sometimes they refer to the large intestine, sometimes to the intestines in general.

The peritoneum is a serous membrane that forms the lining of the abdominal cavity; it covers and supports most of the viscera within the abdomen, and carries the blood and lymph vessels that serve them, as well as the nerves. The term is actually derived from the prefix *peri-* ("around") and the base TON- ("stretching"), but we can think of it as a base in its own right:

3. **PERITON—peritoneum**
   PERITONE—peritoneum

   peritoneal (PERITON-eal) – pertaining to the peritoneum

   pseudoperitonitis (PSEUD-O-PERITON-itis) – inflammation of the peritoneum that is false, i.e., a neurosis in which the symptoms mimic those of peritonitis

   peritoneocentesis (PERITONE-O-centesis) – surgical puncturing of the peritoneum

A large, apronlike fold of peritoneum hangs down from the stomach, covering the intestines; it is called the greater omentum (the lesser omentum, another fold of peritoneum, hangs down from the liver):

4. **OMENT—membrane, omentum**

   omental (OMENT-al) – pertaining to the omentum

   omentorrhaphy (OMENT-O-rrhaphy) – surgical suture of the omentum

   omentosplenopexy (OMENT-O-SPLEN-O-pexy) – surgical fastening of the spleen and omentum

The omentum is sometimes called the epiploon from the Greek meaning "floating upon," since this folded membrane appears to float upon the intestines:

5. **EPIPLO—epiploon, omentum**

   epiplocele (EPIPLO-cele) – hernia of the omentum

   epiploectomy (EPIPLO-ectomy) – surgical removal of the omentum

There are other membranous extensions of the peritoneum that are called mesenteries (singular mesentery); one, in particular, encircles the small intestines. The term mesentery comes from a combination of the prefix *meso-* and the base ENTER-, literally a "middle intestine." But we can think of MESENTER- as a base:

6. **MESENTER—mesentery, membranous fold**

   mesenteric (MESENTER-ic) – pertaining to a mesentery

   mesenteriorrhaphy (MESENTER-I-O-rrhaphy) – surgical suture of the mesentery

   mesenteriopexy (MESENTER-I-O-pexy) – surgical fastening of (a torn) mesentery

Note how both mesenteriorrhaphy and mesenteriopexy have two combining vowels between the base and the compound suffix.

The small intestine consists of three parts, the duodenum, the jejunum, and the ileum. The term duodenum comes from the Latin word for "in twelves," since the small intestine was measured at about twelve fingerbreadths long. According to Galen, the concept originated with Greek doctors from the time of Alexander the Great who used their own word (*dodeka-daktylon*) for something that was "twelve fingerbreadths long":

7. **DUODEN—duodenum**

    duodenitis (DUODEN-itis) – inflammation of the duodenum

    duodenal (DUODEN-al) – pertaining to the duodenum

    cholecystoduodenostomy (CHOLECYST-O-DUODEN-O-stomy) – making a surgical opening between the duodenum and the gallbladder

8. **JEJUN—jejunum**

    jejunotomy (JEJUN-O-tomy) – surgical cutting of the jejunum

    jejunoplasty (JEJUN-O-plasty) – surgical reshaping of the jejunum

    jejunal (JEJUN-al) – pertaining to the jejunum

The jejunum is the middle part of the small intestine. It was called the "empty intestine" or "fasting intestine"—*jejunum intestinum*—by ancient physicians because, as Galen tells us, it is often empty after death. Eventually, it just became known as the jejunum.

9. **ILE—ileum**

    ileac (ILE-ac) – pertaining to the ileum

    jejunoileitis (JEJUN-O-ILE-itis) – inflammation of the ileum and jejunum

    ileoentectropy (ILE-O-*ent-ec*-TROP-y) – condition of inside outside turning of the ileum, i.e., a turning inside-out of a section of the ileum

The ileum is the final portion of the small intestine. Its function is to complete the absorption of nutrients from digested food. We have already seen terms with two prefixes, and we have seen terms where a base precedes a prefix. In ileoentectropy, these two situations combine, but we can just apply a combination of the methods outlined previously. Leave the base that precedes the prefixes till last, and treat the remaining *prefix-prefix*-BASE-suffix in the normal manner by starting with the suffix, then adding the prefixes (the first prefix followed by the second), then adding in your base. After all this, add in the base that precedes the prefixes.

10. **PLIC—to fold, to pleat**

    plicate (PLIC-ate) – having folds or pleats

    replication (*re*-PLIC-ation) – process of again and again folding, i.e., repeating or copying a process

In anatomy, a plica (plural plicae) is a structure in which there is a folding over of the parts; many membranes form plicae. The inner wall of the small intestine is covered with plicae in the form of wrinkles and folds that increase the surface area available for the absorption of nutrients. While the rugae of the stomach are considered temporary structures, since they can unfold when the stomach needs to expand and can then fold back up when not needed, the plicae in the small intestine are permanent features.

The plicae of the small intestine are lined with thousands of villi (singular villus), hairlike projections that increase even more the total surface area over which absorption can take place. Villi occur throughout the body, especially in relation to mucous membranes:

11. VILL—tuft of hair, villus

villous (VILL-ous) – having tufts of hair, pertaining to villi

villitis (VILL-itis) – inflammation of the villi, i.e., inflammation of a surface that possesses villi (often the placenta)

villiform (VILL-I-form) – having the form of a villus or a tuft of hair

12. CAEC—blind, cecum
CEC—blind, cecum

The chief meaning of this base is "blind," but you will almost certainly never come across it in this sense in a compound term. Since the first section of the large intestine leads off on one side to a closed tube (i.e., to a "blind end"), this portion of the intestine was called the cecum (or caecum, in British spelling; plural ceca or caeca). Any similar bodily structure that terminates in a blind end can also be called a cecum:

cecal (CEC-al) – pertaining to a cecum

cecorrhaphy (CEC-O-rrhaphy) – surgical suture of the cecum

ileocecostomy (ILE-O-CEC-O-stomy) – making a surgical opening between the cecum and the ileum

13. TYPHL—blind, cecum

typhlosis (TYPHL-osis) – condition of being blind

typhlomegaly (TYPHL-O-megaly) – enlargement of the cecum

typhlectasis (TYPHL-ectasis) – dilation of the cecum

The term typhlon also refers to any structure that terminates in a blind end, although it is much less used than the term cecum. Unlike CAEC-/CEC-, you will also find TYPHL- in compound terms where it has the meaning "blind."

14. PEND—to hang, to weigh

dependence (*de*-PEND-ence) – state of hanging from (someone or something), i.e., reliance on someone or something for support

The combination of this base with the prefix *ad-* gives us a combination that means "to hang near" or "to hang upon." We can think of APPEND- as a base (notice how *ad-* assimilates to *ap-* before the letter "p"):

15. APPEND—to hang upon

appendant (APPEND-ant) – pertaining to (something that) hangs upon (something else)

In medical terminology, an appendix is a structure that hangs from, or upon, a larger structure. In the digestive system, the appendix is the blind-ended tube that hangs from the cecum. You may see it referred to as the vermiform appendix (remember, we saw VERM-I-form in previous chapter), because it is worm shaped. You will come across both of the following bases with the meaning "appendix" in compound terms:

APPEND—appendix (usually the vermiform appendix)
APPENDIC—appendix (usually the vermiform appendix)

appendectomy (APPEND-ectomy) – surgical removal of the (vermiform) appendix

appendalgia (APPEND-algia) – painful condition (located around the vermiform) appendix

appendicitis (APPENDIC-itis) – inflammation of the (vermiform) appendix

16. COL—colon, large intestine
COLON—colon, large intestine

colocentesis (COL-O-centesis) – surgical puncturing of the colon

enterocolitis (ENTER-O-COL-itis) – inflammation of the colon and small intestine

colonoscopy (COLON-O-scopy) – process of examining the colon with an instrument

The colon already had this name in the time of Aristotle. Some sources define the colon and the large intestine as being two names for the same thing, while others regard the colon as only part of the large intestine (the other parts being some, or all, of the cecum, rectum, and anal canal).

17. DIVERTICUL—diverticulum

The medical noun diverticulum is actually a compound term made from a prefix, a base and a suffix that we have already met (*di*-VERT-I-culum). Literally a "small apart turning," a diverticulum (plural diverticula) is a small pouch or pocket that branches off a larger organ or cavity. Diverticula are generally, though not always, abnormal features that can be problematic. In the digestive system, diverticula may form in the stomach, colon, and duodenum; they may become infected, may cause obstructions, and can sometimes perforate. We can think of DIVERTICUL- as a base:

diverticulitis (DIVERTICUL-itis) – inflammation of a diverticulum
diverticulosis (DIVERTICUL-osis) – abnormal condition (due to) diverticula
diverticulopexy (DIVERTICUL-O-pexy) – surgical fastening of a diverticulum

18. RECT—straight, straighten

erector (*e*-RECT-or) – thing that out straightens, i.e., a muscle that causes a straightening out, or straightening up, of something

You are most likely to come across this base with the meaning "rectum"; this part of the digestive system, which extends between the sigmoid colon (remember, SIGM-oid means "S shaped," like the Greek letter sigma) and the anal canal, got its name because it is a relatively straight portion of the gastrointestinal tract:

RECT—rectum

pararectal (*para*-RECT-al) – pertaining to beside the rectum
rectostenosis (RECT-O-stenosis) – narrowing of the rectum
rectococcygeal (RECT-O-COCCYG-eal) – pertaining to the coccyx and the rectum

19. PROCT—rectum, anus

proctodynia (PROCT-odynia) – painful condition of the rectum or anus
proctology (PROCT-O-logy) – study of (diseases of) the rectum and anus
aproctia (*a*-PROCT-ia) – condition of without an anus

Though the original Greek meaning of this base was "anus," in modern usage it can also mean "rectum."

20. AN—anus

circumanal (*circum*-AN-al) – pertaining to around the anus
anorectocolonic (AN-O-RECT-O-COLON-ic) – pertaining to the colon, rectum, and anus
anoscopy (AN-O-scopy) – process of examining the anus with an instrument

Be careful not to confuse this base with the prefix *an-*. In most cases, the base AN- is followed by the combining vowel "o," but the prefix *an-* may be followed by a base that begins with "o," so there is the potential for confusion; you may have to rely on context to help you.

21. FAEC—feces, dung
FEC—feces, dung

faecal (FAEC-al) – pertaining to feces
feculent (FEC-ulent) – full of feces

You will also see FAEC-al and FEC-al used like bases:

FAECAL—feces
FECAL—feces

faecaloma (FAECAL-oma) – mass of feces
fecaloid (FECAL-oid) – resembling feces

22. STERC—feces
STERCOR—feces

stercolithic (STERC-O-LITH-ic) – pertaining to a stone of feces, i.e., pertaining to a hard mass of feces in the intestines
stercoraceous (STERCOR-aceous) – pertaining to feces
stercoroma (STERCOR-oma) – mass of feces

Stercus is an alternative, though rarely used, term for feces.

23. SCAT—filth, feces

scatophagy (SCAT-O-phagy) – condition of eating feces or filth
scatology (SCAT-O-logy) – study of feces
scatologia (SCAT-O-LOG-ia) – condition of speech that is filthy, i.e., an uncontrollable use of obscene language

This base has meanings that extend beyond "feces" (i.e., anything unclean or considered dirty or obscene), just like COPR- that we saw in an earlier chapter. Here is another similar base:

24. RHYP—filth, feces
RHYPAR—filth, feces

rhypophagy (RHYP-O-phagy) – condition of eating feces or filth
rhypophobia (RHYP-O-phobia) – abnormal fear of filth

rhyparia (RHYPAR-ia) – condition of filth, i.e., a condition in which foul matter forms on the lips and teeth during fevers

One final base related to feces (who knew there were so many):

25. CHEZ—the passing of feces

hematochezia (HEMAT-O-CHEZ-ia) – condition of passing feces (containing) blood

dyschezia (*dys*-CHEZ-ia) – condition of difficult passing of the feces

You will probably only ever come across this base in this combination, CHEZ-ia, "condition of passing feces."

SOME MORE THINGS TO LEARN

Here are some more bases to learn:

26. RHYTI—wrinkle
RHYTID—wrinkle

rhytiphobia (RHYTI-phobia) – abnormal fear of (getting) wrinkles

rhytidectomy (RHYTID-ectomy) – surgical removal of wrinkles

rhytidosis (RHYTID-osis) – abnormal condition of wrinkles, i.e., more wrinkling than expected for age

You may occasionally come across the following bases meaning "wrinkle," but they are much less common:

27. PHARK—wrinkle
PHARKID—wrinkle

pharkophobia (PHARK-O-phobia) – abnormal fear of (getting) wrinkles

pharkidoscopia (PHARKID-O-SCOP-ia) – condition of viewing wrinkles, i.e., an obsession for checking for wrinkles on the face

You may also find the letter "c" replacing the "k" (PHARC- and PHARCID-).

28. STRI—groove, stripe

striate (STRI-ate) – having grooves or stripes

striation (STRI-ation) – process of (creating) stripes

In anatomy, striae (singular stria) are stripes, bands or streaks that differ in color, texture, or height from the surrounding tissues; the bands commonly called stretch marks that some pregnant women get on their stomachs during pregnancy have the technical term *striae gravidarum*, literally "striae of pregnant women" (remember, we have seen the term gravida meaning pregnant woman previously—gravidarum is just a special plural form).

29. PLEX—interwoven, plaited, complicated

plexodontic (PLEX-ODONT-ic) – pertaining to a tooth with complicated (crown or root formation)

This base, which is related to the base PLIC- that we saw above, carries the sense of something folded over on itself many times, and also, a related idea, something of many parts. You will most likely come across this base in relation to the term plexus (plural plexuses), the name for a structure in the body that is an interwoven network of nerves and blood vessels; plexuses occur throughout the body.

PLEX—plexus

plexal (PLEX-al) – pertaining to a plexus

plexitis (PLEX-itis) – inflammation of a plexus

plexectomy (PLEX-ectomy) – surgical removal of a plexus

The solar plexus, the plexus located in the abdomen, got its name from the fact that the nerve fibers radiate out from the center like the rays of the sun (SOL-ar "pertaining to the sun").

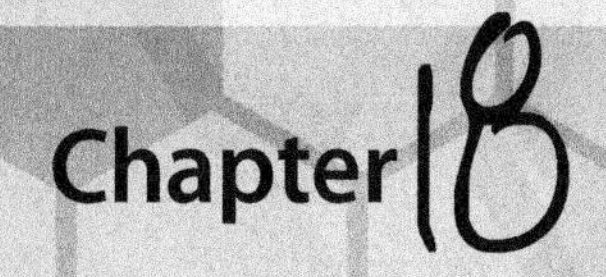

KIDNEYS AND THE BLADDER

We have strayed a little from our head to toe approach since the kidneys are located just below the bottom of the rib cage. They sit, however, posteriorly (i.e., behind) the structures we have already looked at in the abdominal area, in a small area called the retroperitoneal (*retro*-PERITON-eal) space, one on either side of the spine. The right kidney (from the owner's point of view) is slightly lower than the left and sits just below the diaphragm and behind the liver.

BASES

1. **NEPHR—kidney**

   nephrology (NEPHR-O-logy) – study of (diseases of) the kidney

   nephrolithiasis (NEPHR-O-LITH-iasis) – abnormal condition of a stone (or calculus) in the kidney

   laparonephrectomy (LAPAR-O-NEPHR-ectomy) – surgical removal of a kidney through (an incision in) the abdomen

The term laparonephrectomy might seem difficult at first, but if you apply the rules we have learnt (suffix and ultimate base first) we begin with "surgical removal of a kidney." Then we have to apply common sense; it cannot possibly mean "and the abdomen" (abdomens do not get removed), so we think of what is most likely, and "through the abdomen" works fine. In fact, you will find laparo- at the beginning of quite a few terms for medical procedures that are performed through an incision in the abdomen.

2. **REN—kidney**

renal (REN-al) – pertaining to a kidney

renopulmonary (REN-O-PULMON-ary) – pertaining to the lungs and kidneys

renotrophic (REN-O-TROPH-ic) – pertaining to the nutrition of the kidneys

The kidneys are, unsurprisingly, kidneybean-shaped structures (though larger, at about 10 cm long). One of their primary functions is the production of urine that carries waste-products out of the body:

3. **UR—urine**
   URIN—urine

uresis (UR-esis) – process (of passing) urine

urodynia (UR-odynia) – painful condition (when passing) urine

uroscopy (UR-O-scopy) – examination of the urine with an instrument

urinary (URIN-ary) – pertaining to urine

uriniferous (URIN-I-ferous) – pertaining to carrying urine

The combination of the base UR- with the suffix -ia, meaning "condition of the urine," is a common one:

adipuria (ADIP-UR-ia) – condition of the urine (containing) fat

albiduria (ALBID-UR-ia) – condition of the urine (that is) white or pale

hyposthenuria (*hypo*-STHEN-UR-ia) – condition of the urine (whose) strength is less than normal, i.e., a condition in which the urine has a low specific gravity

We can add -uria to our list of compound suffixes. You will also come across the combination of UR- and the suffix -etic:

diuretic (*di*-UR-etic) – pertaining to through (flow) of urine, i.e., pertaining to increased through flow of urine

antidiuretic (*anti-di*-UR-etic) – pertaining to against through (flow) of urine, i.e., pertaining to working against increased through flow of urine

natriuretic (NATR-I-UR-etic) – pertaining to urine (containing) sodium

We can also add -uretic, "pertaining to urine," to our list of compound suffixes.

Closely related to UR- is the base URE- meaning "urea," as well as "urine"; urea is the chief waste product that is excreted in the urine:

4. **URE—urine, urea**

    ureal (URE-al) – pertaining to urea

    ureagenesis (URE-A-genesis) – production of urea

It is not always obvious whether "urine" or "urea" is meant; uresis (URE-sis), for example, generally means "act of producing urine," rather than the production of urea, but in many contexts urine and urea are virtually synonymous, so you probably will not go too far wrong. Another term for producing or passing urine is micturition, but you will probably come across the base MICTUR-, "to pass urine," in only one or two compound terms.

Each of the kidneys has an outer cortex (the CORTIC-al layer); below the cortex is the medulla (MEDULL-ary layer). Urine is collected in cup-shaped structures called calices, or calyces (singular calix or calyx):

5. **CALI—cup-shaped structure, calix**
   CALIC—cup-shaped structure, calix

    caliectasis (CALI-ectasis) – dilation of the (renal) calix

    caliorrhaphy (CALI-O-rrhaphy) – surgical suture of the (renal) calix

    caliceal (CALIC-eal) – pertaining to a calix

    calicectomy (CALIC-ectomy) – surgical removal of a (renal) calix

In turn, the calices drain into the renal pelvis, a funnel-shaped part of the kidney that collects urine.

Here are two bases that both mean "pelvis." The first almost always refers to the renal pelvis, while the second generally, but not always, refers to the basin-shaped collection of bones at the lower end of the vertebral column:

6. **PYEL—renal pelvis, pelvis**

    pyelophlebitis (PYEL-O-PHLEB-itis) – inflammation of the veins of the renal pelvis

    pyelostomy (PYEL-O-stomy) – making a surgical opening in the renal pelvis

    pyelocaliceal (PYEL-O-CALIC-eal) – pertaining to the calices and the renal pelvis

Sometimes PYEL- is combined with NEPHR- to emphasize that it is the pelvis in the kidney (i.e., the renal pelvis) that is meant:

    pyelonephritis (PYEL-O-NEPHR-itis) – inflammation of the kidney pelvis, i.e., inflammation of the renal pelvis

Be careful not to confuse the base PYEL- with the base PY- meaning "pus."

7. **PELV—pelvis, renal pelvis**

    pelvisacral (PELV-I-SACR-al) – pertaining to the sacrum and the pelvis

    pelvicephalometry (PELV-I-CEPHAL-O-metry) – process of measuring the (fetal) head (in relation to the maternal) pelvis

    pelvilithotomy (PELV-I-LITH-O-tomy) – surgical cutting of a stone (via the) renal pelvis, i.e., surgical removal of a kidney stone or calculus through an incision in the renal pelvis

The basic functional units of the kidney are the nephrons, structures that are responsible for filtering the blood that arrives at the kidneys via the renal arteries. Contained within each nephron are the ball-shaped glomerular capsule and the glomerulus (plural glomeruli):

8. **GLOB—ball, ball shaped**
    GLOM—ball shaped
    GLOMER—ball shaped

    globule (GLOB-ule) – small ball, i.e., small spherical body of some kind

    globin (GLOB-in) – substance (that is) ball shaped

    glomal (GLOM-al) – pertaining to a ball-shaped structure, i.e., pertaining to a glomus

    glomerulus (GLOMER-ulus) – small ball-shaped (structure)

The globins are a group of globular (i.e., ball-shaped) proteins; hemoglobin (HEM-O-GLOB-in) is the protein carried by the red blood cells that is responsible for the transport of oxygen. The globulins, also a group of globular proteins, are found only in the blood plasma. A glomus (plural glomera) is a small ball-shaped structure within the body; some glomera act as shunts for blood flow between arterioles and venules. Glomeruli are also small ball-shaped structures; they are often clusters of intertwining capillaries. We can think of GLOMERUL- as a base:

9. **GLOMERUL—glomerulus**

    glomerular (GLOMERUL-ar) – pertaining to a glomerulus

    glomerulonephritis (GLOMERUL-O-NEPHR-itis) – inflammation of the kidney glomerulus

    glomerulopathy (GLOMERUL-O-pathy) – disease of the glomerulus

    glomerulosclerosis (GLOMERUL-O-SCLER-osis) – condition of hardening of the glomerulus (generally the renal glomerulus)

Urine is carried from the renal pelvis to the bladder by two thin tubes about 25 cm long; these structures are the ureters:

10. URETER—ureter

ureteral (URETER-al) – pertaining to the ureter

pyeloureterectasis (PYEL-O-URETER-ectasis) – dilation of the ureter and renal pelvis

hydroureteronephrosis (HYDR-O-URETER-O-NEPHR-osis) – abnormal condition of the kidney and ureter (caused by) fluid, i.e., condition of the kidneys and ureters caused by retained urine

The term hydroureteronephrosis is readily broken down using the method suggested earlier, that is always starting with the suffix and ultimate base, then adding the other bases from right to left (or end to start, if you prefer), and finally adding in whatever words are necessary to make sense. However, you are just as likely to see the term in the form ureterohydronephrosis (URETER-O-HYDR-O-NEPHR-osis), so do be aware that, as always, sometimes common sense has to help out any rules we learn.

11. VESIC—urinary bladder, bladder

vesical (VESIC-al) – pertaining to a bladder

vesicoumbilical (VESIC-O-UMBILIC-al) – pertaining to the umbilicus and the urinary bladder

vesicoclysis (VESIC-O-clysis) – irrigation of the urinary bladder

abdominovesical (ABDOMIN-O-VESIC-al) – pertaining to the urinary bladder and the abdomen, or pertaining to the gallbladder and the abdomen

A bladder can be any hollow structure filled with gas or fluid; the base VESIC- almost always refers to the urinary bladder, but not always. Remember, we saw the base CYST- previously which can mean "bladder," "cyst," or "sac." A vesicula (plural vesiculae) is a small bladder, or bladderlike structure:

vesicula (VESIC-ula) – small bladder

Vesicula can also be the term for a blister, since a blister is just a small structure filled with fluid. You will also come across this term in its anglicized form, vesicle. We can think of VESICUL- as a base:

12. VESICUL—vesicle, small bladder

vesicular (VESICUL-ar) – pertaining to a vesicle

vesiculotomy (VESICUL-O-tomy) – surgical cutting of a vesicle

13. **URETHR—urethra**

   urethrovesicopexy (URETHR-O-VESIC-O-pexy) – surgical fastening of the urinary bladder and urethra

   urethrocystitis (URETHR-O-CYST-itis) – inflammation of the (urinary) bladder and the urethra

   urethrorrhea (URETHR-O-rrhea) – discharge from the urethra

The urethra carries urine from the bladder to the outside of the body; it is longer in men, passing through the prostate gland and the penis.

SOME MORE THINGS TO LEARN

The adrenal (*ad*-REN-al) glands (sometimes called the suprarenal glands) lie on top of the kidneys, one gland on each kidney, but they have nothing to do with the urinary system. They are part of the endocrine system that is responsible for secreting hormones to regulate various bodily functions. Remember, we looked at the terms endocrine and exocrine previously. We can think of ADREN- and ADRENAL- as bases:

14. **ADREN—adrenal gland**
   ADRENAL—adrenal gland

   adrenic (ADREN-ic) – pertaining to an adrenal gland

   adrenocortical (ADREN-O-CORTIC-al) – pertaining to the cortex (outer layer) of the adrenal gland

   adrenalectomy (ADRENAL-ectomy) – surgical removal of an adrenal gland

   adrenalopathy (ADRENAL-O-pathy) – disease of the adrenal gland

The glands that make up the endocrine system are located throughout the body (brain, neck, chest, abdomen, and groin), and some have other functions in other bodily systems. We have already come across the hypothalamus, the pituitary gland, the thyroid glands (also, four parathyroid glands that lie beside the thyroid gland), the thymus, and the pancreas, and we will look at the testes and ovaries in two later chapters. Here are some other bases that relate to the endocrine system:

15. **HYPOPHYS—pituitary gland**

This base is really the prefix *hypo-* and the base PHYS- combined meaning, literally, "undergrowth": hypophysis is an alternative name for the pituitary, the gland that grows under the brain, suspended from the hypothalamus. We will treat HYPOPHYS- as a base:

posthypophysial (*post*-HYPOPHYS-ial) – pertaining to behind the pituitary gland
hypophysitis (HYPOPHYS-itis) – inflammation of the pituitary gland

16. PINE—pinecone

pineal (PINE-al) – pertaining to a pinecone

The pineal gland, or pineal body as it is sometimes called, lies between two lobes of the thalamus; it got its name because its shape resembles a tiny pinecone. One of its functions is secreting hormones related to maintaining biological rhythms such as sleep. We will treat PINEAL- as a base:

17. PINEAL—pineal gland

pinealopathy (PINEAL-O-pathy) – disease of the pineal gland
pinealoma (PINEAL-oma) – tumor of the pineal gland

18. HORMON—hormone

hormonal (HORMON-al) – pertaining to hormones
hormonopoiesis (HORMON-O-poiesis) – formation of hormones
hormonotherapy (HORMON-O-therapy) – treatment with hormones

Hormones were only identified in the 20th century. They took their name from a Greek word meaning "to set in motion," since they act as chemical messengers that set in motion chains of events in the body.

Finally, here are the new compound suffixes we saw in this chapter:

1. -uria	condition of the urine
2. -uretic	pertaining to urine

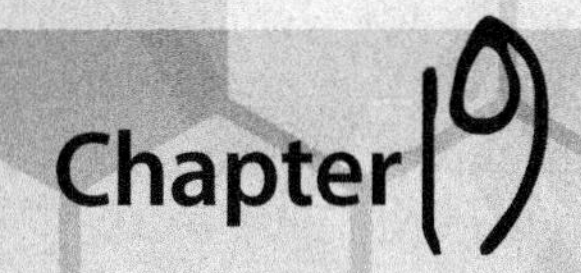

Chapter 19

FEMALE REPRODUCTIVE PARTS

BASES

1. **UTER—uterus, womb**

   uteroabdominal (UTER-O-ABDOMIN-al) – pertaining to the abdomen and uterus

   uterine (UTER-ine) – pertaining to the uterus

   uterosacral (UTER-O-SACR-al) – pertaining to the sacrum and uterus

2. **HYSTER—uterus, womb**

   hysterectomy (HYSTER-ectomy) – surgical removal of the uterus

   hysterocystopexy (HYSTER-O-CYST-O-pexy) – surgical fastening of the (urinary) bladder and the uterus (to the abdominal wall)

   hysterotrachelorrhaphy (HYSTER-O-TRACHEL-O-rrhaphy) – surgical suture of the neck of the uterus

3. **METR—(i) measurement: (ii) uterus, womb**

   metrical (METR-ical) pertaining to measurement

   metrophlebitis (METR-O-PHLEB-itis) – inflammation of the veins of the uterus

   metromalacia (METR-O-malacia) – softening of the uterus (tissues)

   endometrial (*endo*-METR-ial) – pertaining to inside the uterus, i.e., pertaining to the inner layer of the uterine wall

We have already seen this base when we looked at the meaning "measurement." The medical term for the inner layer of the uterine wall is the endometrium; sometimes the endometrial tissue begins to grow outside of the uterus, resulting in a painful condition called endometriosis (*endo*-METR-I-osis).

Here is one rarely used base that means "uterus":

4. DELPH—uterus, womb

didelphic (DI-DELPH-ic) – pertaining to the uterus—two (of them), i.e., pertaining to having a double uterus

5. GONAD—gonad

The gonads are the organs that produce the sex cells, i.e., sperm or eggs. In males, the testes are the gonads, while in females the ovaries fulfill this function.

agonadal (*a*-GONAD-al) – pertaining to (being) without gonads

gonadopathy (GONAD-O-pathy) – disease of the gonads

amphigonadism (*amphi*-GONAD-ism) – condition of (having) both gonads, i.e., having both ovaries and testes, or both ovarian and testicular tissues

The term gonad is a relatively recent introduction formed on the base GON-, meaning "seed":

6. GON—seed

gonocyte (GON-O-cyte) – cell (that forms) seed, i.e., a sperm cell or egg cell

Since the discharge that occurred in certain inflammations of the genital tract resembled a discharge of semen (i.e., discharge of "seed"), the condition was given the name gonorrhea:

gonorrhea (GON-O-rrhea) – flow of seed, i.e., infection with a semenlike discharge

It was many centuries later that the bacterium responsible for the infection was discovered; one of its names is *gonococcus*, so a gonococcicide (GON-O-COCC-I-cide) is a substance that kills the *gonococcus* bacterium.

7. OV—egg

ovoid (OV-oid) – shaped like an egg

ovogenesis (OV-O-genesis) – production of eggs

This base has given rise to several related terms; ovum (egg, the female reproductive cell, plural ova), ovule (OV-ule, "small egg," the female reproductive cell in an early stage), ovary (the reproductive structure that contains the ova), and oviduct (OV-I-duct, the tube linking the ovary to the uterus). We will treat them here as bases:

OV—ovum

ovicide (OV-I-cide) – substance that kills the ovum

oviferous (OV-I-ferous) – pertaining to carrying ova

8. OVUL—ovule

ovular (OVUL-ar) – pertaining to an ovule

ovulogenous (OVUL-O-genous) – pertaining to producing, or being produced by, an ovule

9. OVAR—ovary
OVARI—ovary

ovaritis (OVAR-itis) – inflammation of an ovary

ovariocele (OVARI-O-cele) – hernia of an ovary

ovariopathy (OVARI-O-pathy) – disease of the ovary

10. OVIDUCT—oviduct

oviductal (OVIDUCT-al) – pertaining to an oviduct

oviductitis (OVIDUCT-itis) – inflammation of an oviduct

11. OO—egg

oology (OO-logy) – study of eggs

oophagia (OO-phagia) – condition of eating eggs (habitually)

Like the base OV-, you will most likely come across this base with the specialized meaning ovum:

OO—ovum

oogenic (OO-genic) – producing ova

The related base OOPHOR- (literally, "carrying the ovum") is another base with the meaning "ovary":

12. OOPHOR—ovary

oophorocystectomy (OOPHOR-O-CYST-ectomy) – surgical removal of a cyst on the ovary

oophoropexy (OOPHOR-O-pexy) – surgical fastening of an ovary

oophoralgia (OOPHOR-algia) – painful condition of the ovary

The oviducts are also called uterine tubes and Fallopian tubes (after the first anatomist, Fallopius, who described them correctly).

13. TUB—tube

tubal (TUB-al) - pertaining to a tube

intubation (*in*-TUB-ation) - process of in(serting) a tube (into the body)

tubule (TUB-ule) - a small tube

While there are many tubes, or tubular structures, within the body, this base is sometimes used specifically about the uterine tube:

TUB—uterine tube

tuboabdominal (TUB-O-ABDOMIN-al) - pertaining to the abdomen and uterine tube

tubouterine (TUB-O-UTER-ine) - pertaining to the uterus and uterine tube

Tubes are hollow, cylindrical structures, and the term tube comes originally from a word that means a hollow musical instrument, like a war trumpet. Another term for a hollow, cylindrical structure (i.e., a tube) within the body is salpinx, and this, too, comes from a word meaning a trumpet. You will not come across the word salpinx (plural salpinges) very often, but you will find the base SALPING- in quite a few compound terms, usually relating to the uterine tubes, or to the auditory tube of the ear; you will have to rely on context to help you decide which is most likely:

14. SALPING—tube, uterine tube, auditory tube

salpingopharyngeal (SALPING-O-PHARYNG-eal) - pertaining to the pharynx and auditory tube

salpingocele (SALPING-O-cele) - hernia of a uterine tube

salpingorrhagia (SALPING-O-rrhagia) - excessive discharge from a uterine tube

salpingemphraxis (SALPING-emphraxis) - obstruction of a uterine tube or the auditory tube

15. VAGIN—vagina

vaginovesical (VAGIN-O-VESIC-al) - pertaining to the urinary bladder and the vagina

vaginolabial (VAGIN-O-LABI-al) - pertaining to the labia and the vagina

supravaginal (*supra*-VAGIN-al) - pertaining to above the vagina

cervicovaginitis (CERVIC-O-VAGIN-itis) - inflammation of the vagina and the neck (of the uterus)

The vagina extends from the uterus to the external genitalia. The original meaning for vagina is "sheath" or "scabbard," that is the cover used for a blade or sword. So the term evaginate (*e*-VAGIN-ate) means, literally, "to take (the sword) out of the sheath"; it has come to have the sense of something out of its normal place and to have the medical meaning of "turned inside out" or "protruding out of the normal position." Remember, we saw the base LABI-, meaning "lip," and the term labium, a "liplike structure," previously; two pairs of labia are located alongside the vagina. We have also seen the base CERVIC-, "neck," previously and we noted that the term "neck" is applied to many body parts that have a constricted or narrowed portion. The medical name for the neck of the uterus is the cervix.

16. COLP—vagina

colpomycosis (COLP-O-MYC-osis) – condition of fungal (infection) of the vagina

colpoptosis (COLP-O-ptosis) – prolapse of the vagina

hysterocolpectomy (HYSTER-O-COLP-ectomy) – surgical removal of the vagina and uterus

You might occasionally see this base with the letter "k" replacing the letter "c" (KOLP-).

17. CLITOR—clitoris
CLITORID—clitoris

clitoral (CLITOR-al) – pertaining to the clitoris

clitoromegaly (CLITOR-O-megaly) – enlargement of the clitoris

clitoridectomy (CLITORID-ectomy) – surgical removal of the clitoris

18. VULV—vulva

vulvar (VULV-ar) – pertaining to the vulva

vulvovaginitis (VULV-O-VAGIN-itis) – inflammation of the vagina and vulva

vulvectomy (VULV-ectomy) – surgical removal of the vulva (or part of it)

The external female genitalia, including the labia and the clitoris, are collectively called the vulva. You may also find them called the pudenda (singular pudendum) meaning, literally, "things to be ashamed of."

19. EPISI—vulva

episiostenosis (EPISI-O-stenosis) – narrowing of the vulva (opening)

episioplasty (EPISI-O-plasty) – surgical reshaping of the vulva

20. PERINE—perineum

perineocele (PERINE-O-cele) – hernia in the perineum (area)

episioperineorrhaphy (EPISI-O-PERINE-O-rrhaphy) – surgical suture of the perineum and vulva

In women, the area between the anus and the vulva is termed the perineum. In men, the perineum is the area between the anus and the scrotum.

21. MEN—month, menses

Since the bleeding from the uterus that precedes ovulation occurs, roughly, every month, it got the name menses (literally, the "monthlies," singular mensis) in ancient Greek and Roman times:

menorrhagia (MEN-O-rrhagia) – excessive flow of the menses

menoxenia (MEN-O-XEN-ia) – condition of foreign or strange menses, i.e., condition of abnormal menses

dysmenorrhea (*dys*-MEN-O-rrhea) – flow of difficult menses, i.e., difficult or painful flow of the menses

oligomenorrhea (OLIG-O-MEN-O-rrhea) – flow of menses that is scanty

The base MENSTRU- is related to the base MEN-:

22. MENSTRU—menses

menstruation (MENSTRU-ation) – process of (discharge) of the menses

premenstrual (*pre*-MENSTRU-al) – pertaining to before the menses, i.e., pertaining to before menstruation

postmenstrual (*post*-MENSTRU-al) – pertaining to after the menses, i.e., pertaining to after menstruation

23. ISCH—to suppress

ischomenia (ISCH-O-MEN-ia) – condition of the menses being suppressed

ischemia (ISCH-emia) – condition of blood suppression, i.e., suppression of the blood flow due to an obstruction

ischesis (ISCH-esis) – abnormal condition of suppression (of any discharge)

24. CAPT—to take, to receive
-CEPT—to take, to receive

capture (CAPT-ure) – act of taking

conception (*con*-CEPT-ion) – act of together receiving, i.e., the act of bringing things or ideas together

Note that the form -CEPT- never occurs at the beginning of a term. In medical terminology, conception most often refers to the successful bringing together of sperm and egg. The term contraception (*contra*-CEPT-ion) is actually a shortened form of contraconception (*contra-con*-CEPT-ion), literally "act against together receiving," i.e., against conception. Notice that, in building up this last term, we followed the regular format of suffix-*first prefix-second prefix*-BASE.

25. EMBRY—embryo
EMBRYON—embryo

embryoblast (EMBRY-O-blast) – immature cell (mass inside) the embryo

embryology (EMBRY-O-logy) – study of the embryo, i.e., the study of the development of the embryo

embryomorphous (EMBRY-O-MORPH-ous) – pertaining to the form or shape of the embryo

polyembryonic (POLY-EMBRYON-ic) – pertaining to embryos—many of them, i.e., pertaining to two or more embryos developing from a single fertilized egg

In human medical terminology, we generally use the term embryo for the developing off-spring in the phase between conception and about eight weeks. After eight weeks, and up until the time of birth, the offspring is usually termed a fetus:

26. FET—offspring, fetus
FOET—offspring, fetus

foetal (FOET-al) – pertaining to a fetus

fetometry (FET-O-metry) – process of measuring the fetus

fetation (FET-ation) – process of offspring (formation), i.e., pregnancy

superfetation (*super*-FET-ation) – process of beyond (usual) offspring, i.e., pregnancy involving more than one offspring

You will likely come across both forms of this base, FET- and FOET- (and fetus and foetus). Superfetation is a rare occurrence in human females in which two fetuses are conceived in different menstrual cycles, resulting in two fetuses of different ages.

27. AMNI—amnion
AMNION—amnion

amniotic (AMNI-O-tic) – pertaining to the amnion

amniocentesis (AMNI-O-centesis) – surgical puncturing of the amnion (for sampling of fluid)

amniochorionic (AMNI-O-CHORION-ic) – pertaining to the chorion and the amnion

amnionic (AMNION-ic) – pertaining to the amnion

The amnion is the innermost of the two membranes that surround the fetus, while the chorion is the outer layer (remember, we saw the base CHORI-, CHORION-, CHOROID- earlier; the choroid is a membrane within the eye).

28. PROL—offspring

proligerous (PROL-I-GER-ous) – pertaining to producing offspring

prolific (PROL-I-fic) – making offspring

The meaning "offspring" does not always mean children; it can indicate things produced that are identical to one another, especially in large numbers:

proliferation (PROL-I-FER-ation) – process of producing offspring, i.e., production of similar cells, usually in large numbers

myeloproliferative (MYEL-O-PROL-I-FER-ative) – tending to produce offspring of the bone marrow, i.e., proliferation of the cells of the bone marrow

29. PARTUR—to give birth, childbirth

parturition (PARTUR-I-tion) – process of giving birth

parturifacient (PARTUR-I-facient) – causing childbirth, i.e., inducing labour

parturient (PARTUR-I-ent) – pertaining to childbirth

30. PAR—to give birth

parity (PAR-ity) – condition of giving birth

parous (PAR-ous) – pertaining to giving birth

multiparous (MULT-I-PAR-ous) – pertaining to giving birth many (times)

Remember, we have seen the terms para and gravida previously, meaning "woman who has given birth" and "woman who is/has been pregnant," respectively.

31. CYE—pregnancy

cyesis (CYE-sis) – condition of pregnancy

paracyesis (*para*-CYE-sis) – condition of abnormal pregnancy, i.e., an ectopic pregnancy

acyesis (*a*-CYE-sis) – condition of without pregnancy, i.e., an inability to become pregnant

32. TOC—childbirth
TOK—childbirth

tocology (TOC-O-logy) – study of childbirth

dystocia (*dys*-TOC-ia) – condition of difficult childbirth

bradytokia (BRADY-TOK-ia) – condition of childbirth (that is) slow

Remember, we saw the bases NASC- and NAT-, meaning "being born, birth," previously.

33. PLACENT—placenta

placental (PLACENT-al) – pertaining to the placenta

fetoplacental (FET-O-PLACENT-al) – pertaining to the placenta and the fetus

placentotherapy (PLACENT-O-therapy) – treatment with the placenta, i.e., treatment with the extract of placental tissue

In Latin, *placenta* means a flat, round cake; the organ that connects the fetus to the wall of the uterus, since it is largely flat and round, was given the name placenta. The placenta, along with the ruptured amnion and chorion, is expelled from the body shortly after a woman has given birth. In everyday language, these are collectively called the afterbirth, but you will also see the afterbirth called the secundines, literally the "following things" or "things coming second"; remember, we saw the base SECUND- previously. In the weeks following childbirth, remnants of tissue, blood and mucus are expelled in the lochia:

34. LOCHI- related to childbirth, lochia

lochiorrhea (LOCHI-O-rrhea) – discharge of the lochia

lochiometritis (LOCHI-O-METR-itis) – inflammation of the uterus (due to retained) lochia

lochiostasis (LOCHI-O-stasis) – stoppage of the lochia, i.e., retention of the lochia

35. OBSTETR—obstetrix, midwife

obstetric (OBSTETR-ic) – related to (the duties of the) midwife

This base is derived from the Latin term for a midwife, *obstetrix* (literally, the "one who stands in front"). Its meaning has been extended to include the things that a midwife must deal with, so pregnancy and childbirth:

OBSTETR—pregnancy and childbirth

obstetrics (OBSTETR-ics) – study of pregnancy and childbirth

obstetrician (OBSTETR-ician) – specialist in pregnancy and childbirth

Remember, we saw the base GYNEC-/GYNAEC- previously, meaning "woman"; the specialist that is often referred to by the abbreviation OB/GYN is an obstetrician/gynecologist (or, sometimes the abbreviation refers to the speciality, obstetrics/gynecology).

SOME MORE THINGS TO LEARN

Here are some more bases to learn:

36. MATERN—mother
MATR—mother

matricide (MATR-I-cide) – killing (one's own) mother

maternal (MATERN-al) – pertaining to a mother

maternity (MATERN-ity) – condition of (being) a mother

37. PATERN—father
PATR—father

patricide (PATR-I-cide) – killing (one's own) father

paternal (PATERN-al) – pertaining to a father

paternity (PATERN-ity) – condition of (being) a father

38. FRATERN—brother
FRATR—brother

fratricide (FRATR-I-cide) – killing (one's own) brother

fraternal (FRATERN-al) – pertaining to a brother

Fraternal twins are formed by two separate eggs fertilized by two separate sperm; they are not identical twins.

39. SOROR—sister

sororicide (SOROR-I-cide) – killing (one's own) sister

sororial (SOROR-ial) – pertaining to a sister

The meanings of FRATERN- and SOROR- have been extended to include "close associates" in everyday terms such as fraternity and sorority.

40. TRE—opening
TRES—opening

tresis (TRE-sis) – act of making an opening

atresia (*a*-TRES-ia) – condition of without an opening, i.e., the absence of a normal opening

Vaginal atresia can be a congenital defect (i.e., present at birth), or it can result from the walls of the vagina growing or adhering together. Atresia can occur in many tubelike parts of the body such as the esophagus, intestine, and anus, but also in smaller channels in the heart and pupil of the eye. You will come across the form ATRET- meaning "without an opening." It really is the prefix *a*-, meaning "without," and the base TRET-, "opening," but we will treat it here as a base in its own right:

41. ATRET—without an opening

atretocystia (ATRET-O-CYST-ia) – condition of the (urinary) bladder without an opening

atretogastria (ATRET-O-GASTR-ia) – condition of the stomach without an opening

atretopsia (ATRET-opsia) – condition of sight without an opening, i.e., condition of the pupil of the eye without an opening

42. NE—new, recent

neonatal (NE-O-NAT-al) – pertaining to birth that is recent, i.e., pertaining to immediately after birth

neophobia (NE-O-phobia) – abnormal fear of new (things or events)

neostomy (NE-O-stomy) – making a surgical opening that is new

43. ARCH—ancient, primitive, beginning
ARCHAE—ancient, primitive, beginning
ARCHE—ancient, primitive, beginning

archeocyte (ARCHE-O-cyte) – cell of primitive (form)

archaeocerebellar (ARCHAE-O-CEREBELL-ar) – pertaining to the cerebellum (that evolved) at a primitive (time)

ARCHE- and ARCHAE- are the North American and British spellings of this base. You will rarely see ARCH- at the beginning of a word other than in the term archenteron, the primitive alimentary canal in the embryo. You will, however, see it at the end of a word, combined with the suffix -e that has no meaning; we can think of -arche as a compound suffix meaning "beginning" or "onset":

menarche (MEN-arche) – onset of the menses

44. PALAE—old, primitive
PALE—old, primitive

palaeopathology (PALAE-O-PATH-O-logy) – study of disease in primitive (times)

paleocerebellar (PALE-O-CEREBELL-ar) – pertaining to the cerebellum (that evolved) at a primitive (time)

Again, PALAE- and PALE- are just the alternative North American and British spellings of this base.

45. CHRON—time

chronometry (CHRON-O-metry) – process of measuring time (or intervals of time)

chronograph (CHRON-O-graph) – instrument used to record time (or intervals of time)

chronic (CHRON-ic) – pertaining to time, i.e., lasting a long time in relation to illness and disease

Finally, here is the new compound suffix we saw in this chapter:

1	-arche	beginning, onset

Chapter 20

MALE REPRODUCTIVE PARTS

BASES

1. **TEST—testis**

    testalgia (TEST-algia) – painful condition of a testis

    testopathy (TEST-O-pathy) – disease of a testis

    testectomy (TEST-ectomy) – surgical removal of a testis

The primary meaning of the Latin word testis (plural testes) is "witness," as in testimony or testify, but, for some reason that no one is quite sure of, the same word was applied to the male gonad. The term testicle is actually derived from a diminutive form:

testiculus (TEST-I-culus) – small testis, i.e., a testicle

In medical terminology, the two terms, testis and testicle, mean exactly the same. We can think of TESTICUL- as a base:

2. **TESTICUL—testicle, testis**

    testicular (TESTICUL-ar) – pertaining to a testicle

    testiculitis (TESTICUL-itis) – inflammation of a testicle

3. **ORCH—testis**
   ORCHI—testis
   ORCHID—testis

   cryptorchism (CRYPT-ORCH-ism) – condition of the testis (being) hidden, i.e., condition of the testis failing to descend into the scrotum

   orchioplasty (ORCHI-O-plasty) – surgical reshaping of a testis

   orchidoptosis (ORCHID-O-ptosis) – prolapse of a testis

   cryptorchidectomy (CRYPT-ORCHID-ectomy) – surgical removal of a testis (that is) hidden, i.e., surgical removal of an undescended testis

Though you will rarely come across the term orchis (plural orchises) for the male gonad (testis is the preferred name), the related bases are used frequently in compound medical terms. Orchid plants got their name because their roots (supposedly) resemble testes.

4. **DIDYM—(i) twin: (ii) testis**

   didymodynia (DIDYM-odynia) – painful condition of a testis

   didymitis (DIDYM-itis) – inflammation of a testis

The earliest meaning of this term was "double" or "twofold." This was later extended to include "twin," and then, even later, "testis" or "testicle." The medical term didymus is used about a single testis; you will probably never see the plural form, which is didymoi. Sometimes, you will come across the form -didymus at the end of a word acting like a suffix; it generally has the meaning "twin," or "conjoined twins." You will not see it a lot, which is good, because it can be a bit tricky:

cephalodidymus (CEPHAL-O-didymus) – conjoined twins (fused everywhere except the) head

thoracodidymus (THORAC-O-didymus) – conjoined twins (fused at the) thorax

cryptodidymus (CRYPT-O-didymus) – twin (that is) hidden, i.e., a poorly developed twin that is concealed within the larger one

You are more likely to come across the form -pagus in compound terms relating to sets of conjoined twins; it is connected to the base PEX- ("to fasten") that we have already seen, and it always indicates the place at which a set of conjoined twins are fused together:

craniopagus (CRANI-O-pagus) – conjoined twins (fused at the) cranium

thoracogastropagus (THORAC-O-GASTR-O-pagus) – conjoined twins (fused at the) stomach and thorax

omphalopagus (OMPHAL-O-pagus) – conjoined twins (fused at the) navel

We can add -didymus and -pagus to our list of compound suffixes.

Getting back to the meaning "testis," the epididymis (plural epididymides) is a narrow, tightly-coiled tube that sits on the surface of the testis (remember, *epi-* "on the surface"). We can think of EPIDIDYM- as a base:

5. EPIDIDYM—epididymis

epididymotomy (EPIDIDYM-O-tomy) – surgical cutting of the epididymis

epididymoplasty (EPIDIDYM-O-plasty) – surgical reshaping of the epididymis

orchiepididymitis (ORCH-I-EPIDIDYM-itis) – inflammation of the epididymis and the testis

The epididymis is responsible for conveying sperm from the testis to the vas deferens; remember, we looked at the base VAS- ("vessel" or "vas") previously. The testes and associated epididymides are suspended within a sack of skin and muscle, the scrotum:

6. SCROT—scrotum

scrotocele (SCROT-O-cele) – hernia of the scrotum

scrotiform (SCROT-I-form) – like a scrotum, i.e., shaped like a sack or pouch

urethroperineoscrotal (URETHR-O-PERINE-O-SCROT-al) – pertaining to the scrotum, perineum and urethra

7. OSCHE—scrotum

oscheal (OSCHE-al) – pertaining to the scrotum

oscheohydrocele (OSCHE-O-HYDR-O-cele) – swelling (composed of) fluid in the scrotum

oscheitis (OSCHE-itis) – inflammation of the scrotum

8. SEMIN—seed, semen, seminal fluid

While technically the meaning of semen is "seed," its sense has been extended to include seminal fluid, the secretion which is emitted during ejaculation, whether it contains seed (i.e., sperm) or not.

seminal (SEMIN-al) – pertaining to semen

seminiferous (SEMIN-I-ferous) – carrying seed or seminal fluid

insemination (*in*-SEMIN-ation) – process of in(planting) seed, i.e., introduction of semen into the vagina

9. **SPERM—seed, semen, sperm**
   spermicide (SPERM-I-cide) – substance that kills sperm
   spermiduct (SPERM-I-duct) – tube (that carries) sperm
   oligospermia (OLIG-O-SPERM-ia) – condition of sperm being scanty

In medical terminology, the term spermatozoon (plural spermatozoa) is often preferred over sperm:

10. **ZO—animal, living thing**
    protozoic (PROT-O-ZO-ic) – pertaining to living things that are primitive, i.e., pertaining to primitive unicellular organisms
    zoogenesis (ZO-O-genesis) – production of living things

You will often find this base at the end of words in the form -zoon, acting like a suffix meaning "animal" or "living thing"; we will add it to our list of compound suffixes.

11. **SPERMAT—spermatozoon, semen, sperm**
    spermatogenesis (SPERMAT-O-genesis) – production of spermatozoa
    spermatorrhea (SPERMAT-O-rrhea) – (involuntary) discharge of semen
    spermaturia (SPERMAT-uria) – condition of the urine that contains semen

12. **PEN—penis**
    penile (PEN-ile) – pertaining to the penis

Remember, we have already seen another base PEN- meaning "deficiency, decrease." You will only rarely come across this base in compound terms; a more commonly used base meaning penis is PHALL-:

13. **PHALL—penis**
    phallic (PHALL-ic) – pertaining to the penis
    phallocampsis (PHALL-O-CAMP-sis) – condition of a bent penis (during erection)
    phallorrhea (PHALL-O-rrhea) – discharge from the penis

14. **BALAN—(i) acorn: (ii) glans penis**
    balanoid (BALAN-oid) – resembling an acorn
    balanoplasty (BALAN-O-plasty) – surgical reshaping of the glans penis
    balanitis (BALAN-itis) – inflammation of the glans penis

Because of some similarity in shape, the rounded head of the penis (the glans penis) was named from the Greek word for acorn, *balanos*. The foreskin that covers most of the glans penis is called the prepuce; you probably could not guess that the base that means "prepuce" or "foreskin" in compound terms is actually PREPUTI-:

15. PREPUTI—prepuce, foreskin

preputial (PREPUTI-al) – pertaining to the prepuce

parapreputial (*para*-PREPUTI-al) – pertaining to beside the prepuce

preputiotomy (PREPUTI-O-tomy) – surgical cutting of the foreskin

16. PROSTAT—prostate gland

prostatocystitis (PROSTAT-O-CYST-itis) – inflammation of the (urinary) bladder and the prostate gland

prostatorrhea (PROSTAT-O-rrhea) – discharge from the prostate gland

prostatolithotomy (PROSTAT-O-LITH-O-tomy) – surgical cutting of a stone in the prostate gland, i.e., removal of a calculus in the prostate gland

The prostate is a gland located between the bladder and the penis, and both urine and sperm pass through it; it secretes a fluid that both nourishes and protects the sperm.

Here are three bases that relate to the act of intercourse:

17. COIT—sexual intercourse

postcoital (*post*-COIT-al) – pertaining to after sexual intercourse

coitophobia (COIT-O-phobia) – abnormal fear of sexual intercourse

This base gives us the most common medical term for intercourse, coitus.

18. VENERE—sexual intercourse

venereal (VENERE-al) – pertaining to sexual intercourse

This base is derived from the name of the ancient Roman goddess of love, Venus. The term venereal is used largely about diseases transmitted during sexual intercourse:

VENERE—sexually transmitted

venereology (VENERE-O-logy) – study of sexually transmitted (diseases)

venereophobia (VENERE-O-phobia) – abnormal fear of sexually transmitted (diseases)

19. PAREUN—sexual intercourse

pareunia (PAREUN-ia) – act of sexual intercourse

dyspareunia (*dys*-PAREUN-ia) – condition of painful sexual intercourse

SOME MORE THINGS TO LEARN

Prostate cancer is, at the moment, one of the most common of cancers among men. It can be hard to detect at an early stage, but it does generally respond very well to treatment. Here are some bases that refer to cancer and its treatment:

20. CARCIN- (i) crab: (ii) cancer, malignant tumor

carcinomorphic (CARCIN-O-morphic) – pertaining to the form of a crab

carcinoma (CARCIN-oma) – tumor of cancer (cells)

adenocarcinoma (ADEN-O-CARCIN-oma) – tumor of cancer (cells) in a gland

carcinogenic (CARCIN-O-genic) – producing cancer

carcinectomy (CARCIN-ectomy) – surgical removal of a malignant tumor

Hippocrates was the first to use the Greek word for crab, *karkinos*, about malignant tumors. Later writers and physicians suggested various reasons as to what the resemblance was, but we have no record of what Hippocrates himself thought. Whatever it was, the name stuck, and Roman physicians copied the idea and used the Latin word for crab for the tumors and the associated disease; you will probably never across this base with the meaning "crab":

21. CANCER—cancer, malignant tumor
CANCR—cancer, malignant tumor

cancerophobia (CANCER-O-phobia) – abnormal fear of (acquiring) malignant tumors

precancerous (*pre*-CANCER-ous) – pertaining to before cancer, i.e., pertaining to something likely to develop into cancer

cancriform (CANCR-I-form) – having the form of a malignant tumor, or of cancer

22. ONC—mass, tumor

oncology (ONC-O-logy) – study of tumors

oncotherapy (ONC-O-therapy) – treatment of tumors

oncogenic (ONC-O-genic) – producing tumors

Galen preferred the term *onkos*, literally a "mass" or "large body," for malignant tumors. You may find this base at the end of words in the form -oncus, acting like a suffix meaning "tumor" or "swelling":

adenoncus (ADEN-oncus) – swelling of a gland

blepharoncus (BLEPHAR-oncus) – tumor on the eyelid

We will add -oncus to our list of compound suffixes.

23. PHARMAC—drug

pharmacotherapy (PHARMAC-O-therapy) – treatment by drugs

pharmacology (PHARMAC-O-logy) – study of drugs

24. CHEM—chemical

chemoserotherapy (CHEM-O-SER-O-therapy) – treatment with serum and chemicals

polychemotherapy (POLY-CHEM-O-therapy) – treatment with chemicals–many (of them), i.e., treatment with varied chemicals

We have now seen two terms for tumors that use the suffix -oma, namely carcinoma and sarcoma. You will likely come across them at the end of longer compound terms where they indicate the type of tumor involved, -carcinoma indicating a malignant tumor originating in the epithelial cells, -sarcoma indicating a malignant tumor originating in cells of the soft tissues. We have also seen that the term blastoma, and the ending -blastoma, can, likewise, indicate a malignant tumor, but in this case originating in immature cells. Blastomas generally occur in infants. We can think of -carcinoma, -sarcoma, and -blastoma as compound suffixes meaning "malignant tumor." In compound terms, they can indicate the location of the tumor, as in adenocarcinoma, osteosarcoma, and retinablastoma, or the exact type of cells they are made from, as in fibrocarcinoma, lymphosarcoma, and lipoblastoma.

Here is one final base to learn for this chapter:

25. TERAT—monster, teras, malformed

teratogenic (TERAT-O-genic) – producing a monster, i.e., causing a malformed fetus

teratosis (TERAT-osis) – abnormal condition (resulting in) a malformed (fetus)

teratospermia (TERAT-O-SPERM-ia) – condition of sperm being malformed

A fetus that is grossly malformed may be termed a teras, literally a "monster." We also find this base used in oncology:

teratoma (TERAT-oma) – tumor that is a monster, i.e., a tumor made up of diverse tissues

A teratoma is a somewhat bizarre tumor made up of tissues totally unrelated to the organ in which it is found. Teratomas may be malignant, or non-malignant.

Finally, here are the new compound suffixes we saw in this chapter:

1. -blastoma	malignant tumor
2. -carcinoma	malignant tumor
3. -didymus	twin, conjoined twins
4. -oncus	tumor, swelling
5. -pagus	conjoined twins
6. -sarcoma	malignant tumor
7. -zoon	animal, living thing

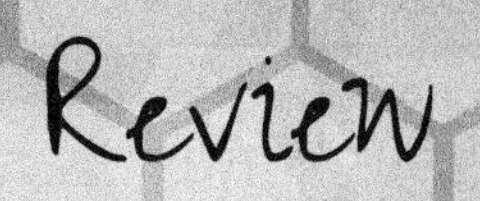

CHAPTERS 16–20

PREFIXES

We did not add any new prefixes to our list.

SUFFIXES

We did not add any new suffixes to our list.

COMPOUND SUFFIXES

We did add some new compound suffixes to our list. Remember, it is helpful to memorize all the compound suffixes because they occur so regularly, but you can also always build them up from their individual base and suffix parts.

Most of the compound suffixes we have made are nouns. Here are the ones that relate to the senses and the mind:

1. -acousia	condition of hearing
2. -blepsia	condition of sight
3. -esthesia	condition of sensation
4. -geusia	condition of sense of taste
5. -mania	condition of madness, compulsion, obsession
6. -mnesia	condition of memory, memory
7. -opia	condition of sight

8. -opsia	condition of sight
9. -osmia	condition of sense of smell
10. -philia	condition of attraction, abnormal craving for
11. -phobia	condition of fear, abnormal fear of

Here are the ones that relate to medical procedures and treatment:

12. -agogue	stimulating, promoting flow of
13. -centesis	surgical puncturing, puncturing
14. -cide	killing, substance that kills
15. -clasia, -clasis	surgical fracture, breaking, rupture
16. -cleisis	surgical closure, closure
17. -clysis	therapeutic infusion of liquid, irrigation
18. -desis	surgical fusion, binding
19. -dialysis	surgical dissolving, surgical separation, filtration
20. -ectomy	surgical removal, removal
21. -fuge	substance that expels, substance that drives away
22. -iatrics, -iatry	medical treatment
23. -lysis	surgical dissolving, surgical separation, loosening
24. -pexis, -pexy	surgical fastening, fixing
25. -plasia, -plasty	surgical reshaping, formation
26. -stat	agent that inhibits, agent that retards
27. -stomy	making a surgical opening, making an opening
28. -therapia, -therapy	treatment
29. -tripsy	surgical crushing, crushing
30. -tomy	surgical cutting, cutting

Here are the ones that express some physical condition:

31. -aemia, -emia	condition of the blood
32. -agra	pain, painful seizure
33. -algesia	sensation of pain
34. -algia	painful condition
35. -asthenia	weakness
36. -atrophia, -atrophy	wasting
37. -blastoma	malignant tumor
38. -carcinoma	malignant tumor
39. -cele	hernia, protrusion, swelling
40. -coel, -coele	cavity
41. -dactylia, -dactyly	condition of the fingers or toes
42. -dystrophia, -dystrophy	weakness
43. -ectasia, -ectasis	expansion, widening, dilation
44. -ectopia, -ectopy	displacement
45. -edema	swelling
46. -emesia, -emesis	vomiting
47. -emphraxis	obstruction
48. -haemia, -hemia	condition of the blood
49. -lepsis, -lepsy	seizure
50. -malacia	softening
51. -megaly	enlargement
52. -nosia	disease
53. -odynia	painful condition
54. -oncus	tumor, swelling
55. -pathia, -pathy	disease, treatment of disease

56. -penia	deficiency
57. -phthisis	wasting
58. -plegia	paralysis
59. -plexia, -plexy	seizure
60. -ptosia, -ptosis	drooping, prolapse
61. -sarcoma	malignant tumor
62. -schisis	fissure
63. -stasia, -stasis, -stasy	stoppage, stagnation
64. -stenosis	narrowing, contraction
65. -syndactylia, -syndactyly	condition of fused fingers or toes
66. -uria	condition of the urine

The -rrh compounds are not true compound suffixes in the way we have described them, but they do occur quite often, so it is good to be aware of them:

67. -rrhage	excessive flow, excessive discharge
68. -rrhagia	excessive flow, excessive discharge
69. -rrhaphy	surgical suture
70. -rrhea	flow, discharge
71. -rrhexis	rupture

Here are the remaining compound suffixes that form nouns:

72. -arche	beginning, onset
73. -blast	immature cell
74. -crine	thing that secretes
75. -cyte	cell

76. -didymus	twin, conjoined twins
77. -genesis	production
78. -graphy	process of recording
79. -gravida	woman who is, or has been, pregnant
80. -logist	one who studies
81. -logy	study of
82. -metry	process of measuring
83. -pagus	conjoined twins
84. -para	woman who has given birth
85. -phage	thing that devours
86. -phagia, -phagy	condition of eating
87. -phyte	plant, growth
88. -pnea	breathing, respiration
89. -poiesis	making, formation
90. -scopy	process of examining with an instrument
91. -tome	instrument used to cut
92. -zoon	animal, living thing

These compound suffixes form adjectives:

93. -facient	making, causing
94. -ferous	bearing, carrying, producing
95. -genic	producing, produced
96. -genous	producing, produced
97. -uretic	pertaining to urine
98. -verse	to turn, to travel, turned

BUILDING UP MEDICAL DEFINITIONS

We did not see any new forms, but we did see a term that combines two of the oddities we had previously encountered. The term ileoentectropy (ILE-O-*ent-ec*-TROP-y) not only has two prefixes, it also has a base preceding a prefix. But we were able to just use a combination of the methods outlined previously. Leave the base that precedes the prefixes till last, and treat the remaining *prefix-prefix*-BASE-suffix in the normal manner by starting with the suffix, then adding the prefixes (the first prefix followed by the second), then adding in your base. After all this, add in the base that precedes the prefixes.

We also encountered a number of terms that have two consecutive combining vowels—portobilioarterial (PORT-O-BIL-I-O-ARTER-ial), mesenteriorrhaphy (MESENTER-I-O-rrhaphy), and mesenteriopexy (MESENTER-I-O-pexy). Again, they did not really present any problem, since combining vowels do not add anything to the definition.

Chapter 21

HIPS AND LEGS

BASES

1. **ILI—upper hip bone, ilium**

   iliococcygeal (ILI-O-COCCYG-eal) – pertaining to the coccyx and ilium

   iliopagus (ILI-O-pagus) – conjoined twins (fused at the) ilium

   sacroiliac (SACR-O-ILI-ac) – pertaining to the ilium and the sacrum

Be careful not to confuse the bases ILE- and ILI-. In the original Latin, the terms *ileum* and *ilium* mean exactly the same, a rather imprecise area somewhere between the abdomen and groin. In modern medical terminology, the term ileum (as we saw previously) is used about a section of the small intestine; the term ilium is used about one of the three major bones that make up the hip bone, the other two being the ischium and the pubis:

2. **ISCHI—lower hip bone, ischium**

   ischialgia (ISCHI-algia) – painful condition of the ischium

   ischiothoracopagus (ISCHI-O-THORAC-O-pagus) – conjoined twins (fused at the) thorax and ischium

   ischiovertebral (ISCHI-O-VERTEBR-al) – pertaining to the spine and ischium

The medical term sciatic is actually a corruption on this base; it is, more correctly, ischiatic, i.e., ISCHI-atic—pertaining to the ischium. Thus, sciatica, a condition involving pain in the hip area that radiates downwards is, more correctly, ischialgia.

3. **PUB—pubic bone, pubis, pubic hair**

    puboprostatic (PUB-O-PROSTAT-ic) – pertaining to the prostate gland and the pubic bone

    puborectal (PUB-O-RECT-al) – pertaining to the rectum and the pubic bone

    suprapubic (*supra*-PUB-ic) – pertaining to above the pubic bone

In compound terms, this base almost always refers to the pubic bone, i.e., the pubis, but you may come across the term pubes (the plural of pubis) meaning the hair that covers the genital regions or, occasionally, the genitals themselves. Here is one compound term where the meaning of the base is pubic hair:

pubarche (PUB-arche) – onset of the pubic hair, i.e., the beginning of puberty

Remember, we saw the base PUBER-/PUBERT- previously.

Together, the ilium, ischium, and pubis make up one hip bone; two hip bones (one left and one right), along with the sacrum and the coccyx, make up the pelvis, a basin-shaped part of the skeleton. We saw the base PELV- previously, and its original meaning is, in fact, "basin"; any basin- or funnel-shaped cavity might be termed a pelvis, as is the renal pelvis of the kidney that we mentioned earlier.

4. **COX—hip bone, hip joint, coxa**

    coxodynia (COX-odynia) – painful condition of the hip joint

    coxotomy (COX-O-tomy) – surgical cutting of the hip bone

    coxotuberculosis (COX-O-TUBERCUL-osis) – abnormal condition (affecting the) tubercles of the hip bone

5. **ACETABUL—hip bone socket, acetabulum**

    acetabular (ACETABUL-ar) – pertaining to the acetabulum

    acetabulectomy (ACETABUL-ectomy) – surgical removal of the acetabulum

The acetabulum is the hollow, cuplike cavity in the pelvis into which the head of the thigh bone fits. The term comes from the Latin word *acetabulum* that is a shallow cup for holding vinegar—remember the base ACET- that we saw previously.

6. **INGUIN—groin**

    inguinal (INGUIN-al) – pertaining to the groin

    inguinoscrotal (INGUIN-O-SCROT-al) – pertaining to the scrotum and groin

    inguinodynia (INGUIN-odynia) – painful condition of the groin

    lumboinguinal (LUMB-O-INGUIN-al) – pertaining to the groin and loin

The term groin generally indicates the area where the thigh meets the trunk of the body.

7. **GLUTE—buttocks**

    gluteoinguinal (GLUTE-O-INGUIN-al) – pertaining to the groin and buttocks

    gluteal (GLUTE-al) – pertaining to the buttocks

8. **PYG—buttocks**

    pygal (PYG-al) – pertaining to the buttocks

    pygopagus (PYG-O-pagus) – conjoined twins (attached at the) buttocks

    steatopygia (STEAT-O-PYG-ia) – condition of the buttocks (with excessive) fat

Clunes and nates are two Latin terms used for the buttocks, but you will rarely see either of their bases used in compound terms.

9. **FEMOR—thigh, femur**

    femoral (FEMOR-al) – pertaining to the thigh or femur

    inguinofemoral (INGUIN-O-FEMOR-al) – pertaining to the femur, or thigh, and the groin

The femur, the longest and strongest bone in the human body, is the only bone within the thigh; sometimes the base FEMOR- refers to the bone itself, sometimes to the thigh (which is its original meaning).

10. **TROCHANTER—trochanter**

    subtrochanteric (*sub*-TROCHANTER-ic) – pertaining to below a trochanter

    trochanterian (TROCHANTER-ian) – pertaining to a trochanter

    trochanterplasty (TROCHANTER-plasty) – surgical reshaping of the trochanter

    trochanteritis (TROCHANTER-itis) – inflammation of the trochanter

Just below the head of the femur (the head is the part that engages with the acetabulum in the pelvis) are two bony projections to which muscles attach; these are the greater (i.e., the bigger) and lesser (i.e., smaller) trochanters.

11. **CRUR—thigh, leg, crus**

    brachiocrural (BRACHI-O-CRUR-al) – pertaining to leg and arm

    intercrural (*inter*-CRUR-al) – pertaining to between the thighs

Crus (plural crura) is generally a medical term used for the leg, or a part of the leg, but it can sometimes be used for a structure that resembles a leg, like a crest or ridge:

    crural (CRUR-al) – pertaining to a crus

12. SCEL—leg
SKEL—leg

scelalgia (SCEL-algia) – painful condition of the leg

macroskelia (MACR-O-SKEL-ia) – condition of the legs that are (abnormally) large

skelasthenia (SKEL-asthenia) – weakness of the legs

You will come across both spellings of this base. It is not related to the term skeleton, which actually comes from the Greek word *skeletos* meaning "dried up" or "withered."

13. GON—knee

gonarthrotomy (GON-ARTHR-O-tomy) – surgical cutting of the joint in the knee

gonocampsis (GON-O-CAMP-sis) – condition of (permanently) bent knee

gonarthritis (GON-ARTHR-itis) – inflammation of the joint in the knee

Remember, we have already seen the base GON- meaning "seed"; luckily, the meanings of the two bases are sufficiently different that the other parts of the compound term usually give a good indication of which base is being used.

14. GEN—knee

genual (GEN-U-al) – pertaining to the knee

genupectoral (GEN-U-PECTOR-al) – pertaining to the chest and knee, i.e., relating to a position resting face forward on knees and upper chest

genucubital (GEN-U-CUBIT-al) – pertaining to the elbow and knee, i.e., relating to a position resting face forward on knees and elbows

geniculum (GEN-I-culum) – a small knee, i.e., a small kneelike structure, one that has a bend in it like the knee joint

Again, we have already seen a base with an identical form, GEN- meaning "to produce." GEN- meaning "knee," however, is almost always followed by the combining vowel "u." In fact, the term genu (plural genua) is sometimes used in medical terminology for the knee, or for a kneelike structure. The term geniculum (plural genicula) is used about a small genu, or a small, kneelike structure such as a sharp bend in an organ or nerve; we can think of GENICUL- as a base:

15. GENICUL—geniculum

genicular (GENICUL-ar) – pertaining to a geniculum

geniculated (GENICUL-ated) – having a geniculum

16. POPLIT—back of the knee

popliteal (POPLIT-eal) – pertaining to the back of the knee
suprapopliteal (*supra*-POPLIT-eal) – pertaining to above the back of the knee
subpopliteal (*sub*-POPLIT-eal) – pertaining to below the back of the knee

The poples is a region at the back of the knee, but you will rarely come across the term.

17. PATELL—kneecap, patella

patellalgia (PATELL-algia) – painful condition of the kneecap
postpatellar (*post*-PATELL-ar) – pertaining to behind the kneecap
infrapatellar (*infra*-PATELL-ar) – pertaining to below the kneecap

The patella is a triangular bone that covers the surface of the knee joint. The original Latin term *patella* means a small dish or small pan (remember the suffix -ella meaning "small"); the underside of the patella bone is slightly concave, so it (sort of) resembles a small dish.

18. MENISC—crescent shaped, meniscus

meniscopexy (MENISC-O-pexy) – surgical fastening of the meniscus
meniscotome (MENISC-O-tome) – instrument used to cut a meniscus
meniscocyte (MENISC-O-cyte) – cell that is crescent shaped, i.e., another term for drepanocyte, the sickle-shaped cell that is characteristic of sickle cell anaemia

A meniscus (plural menisci) is a crescent-shaped structure; the term is linked to the Greek term for "small moon," that is the moon when it is in its crescent form and not a full moon. In the knee, there are two menisci, crescent-shaped pieces of cartilage that disperse friction in the knee joint. Menisci are also present in joints related to the jaw, wrist, and collar bone.

19. TIBI—shin bone, tibia

pretibial (*pre*-TIBI-al) – pertaining to in front of the shin bone
tibiad (TIBI-ad) – toward the tibia
tibiofemoral (TIBI-O-FEMOR-al) – pertaining to the femur and the tibia

The tibia is the larger of the two bones in the lower leg; it is a weight-bearing bone.

20. FIBUL—fibula

fibular (FIBUL-ar) – pertaining to the fibula
tibiofibular (TIBI-O-FIBUL-ar) – pertaining to the fibula and tibia

The fibula is the more slender of the two bones in the lower leg; it does not bear any weight. While the tibia had its name in Roman times, the fibula was only called this much later. In Latin, *fibula* means a fastening or clasp, a sort of safety pin used to hold clothes in position; because the tibia and the fibula together look like a fastening device, the fibula was later given this name. The name for this bone in Latin is *sura*; it also means "calf of the leg," and you may occasionally come across the term sural meaning "pertaining to the calf of the leg," but you are unlikely to see the base SUR- in any other compound terms.

21. CNEM—leg, lower leg
KNEM—leg, lower leg

cnemial (CNEM-ial) – pertaining to the lower leg

brachycnemia (BRACHY-CNEM-ia) – condition of the lower legs that are (abnormally) short

aknemia (*a*-KNEM-ia) – condition of without legs or lower legs, i.e., congenital absence of either the entire leg, or the lower leg

You will see this base with both spellings. Its original meaning relates to the armor that a Greek soldier wore to protect his lower legs, whether leather leggings or metal greaves. Aknemia (or, acnemia) can also mean the loss of the musculature of the lower legs. You will come across this base in what seems like an unusual combination, gastrocnemius. This is the name for the muscle in the calf of the leg; because of its bulging, stomachlike shape, it got the name that it did.

SOME MORE THINGS TO LEARN

Here are some new bases to learn; they do not really relate to hips and legs, other than people often complain of their "legs going to sleep":

22. HYPN—sleep

ahypnia (*a*-HYPN-ia) – condition of without sleep, i.e., a prolonged state without sleep

hypnotherapy (HYPN-O-therapy) – treatment by (prolonged) sleep

hypnagogue (HYPN-agogue) – stimulating sleep

hypnosis (HYPN-osis) – abnormal condition of sleep

The term hypnosis has taken on the special meaning of an intentionally induced, sleeplike state; you may have to rely on context to decide which meaning for HYPN- is intended:

23. HYPN—hypnosis
HYPNOT—hypnosis

hypnotherapy (HYPN-O-therapy) – treatment by hypnosis

hypnodontics (HYPN-ODONT-ics) – science of (treating) teeth along with hypnosis (of the patient), i.e., hypnosis in the practice of dentistry

hypnotic (HYPNOT-ic) – pertaining to hypnosis

24. SOMN—sleep

somnifacient (SOMN-I-facient) – causing sleep

somnipathy (SOMN-I-pathy) – disease of sleep, i.e., a sleep disorder

somniloquist (SOMN-I-LOQU-ist) – person who speaks during sleep

insomnia (*in*-SOMN-ia) – condition of not sleeping

25. NARC—numbness, stupor

narcolepsy (NARC-O-lepsy) – seizure by stupor or numbness

narcotic (NARC-O-tic) – pertaining to the condition of stupor, i.e., a substance that can induce a state of stupor

encephalonarcosis (ENCEPHAL-O-NARC-osis) – abnormal condition of stupor (caused by) brain (disease)

26. ONEIR—dream

oneiric (ONEIR-ic) – pertaining to dreams

oneirodynia (ONEIR-odynia) – painful condition (pertaining to) a dream, i.e., a nightmare

oneirologist (ONEIR-O-logist) – one who studies dreams

27. NYCT—night

nycturia (NYCT-uria) – condition of the urine (being passed frequently) at night

nyctophobia (NYCT-O-phobia) – abnormal fear of the night (or darkness)

nyctanopia (NYCT-*an*-OP-ia) – condition of non-sight at night, i.e., night blindness

Because the term nyctanopia has a prefix preceded by a base, it is actually easier to treat the base OP- and the suffix -ia separately here, rather than as the compound suffix -opia (so, "condition of non-sight" rather than "condition of sight—non").

Chapter 22

FEET AND TOES

BASES

1. TARS—ankle, edge of the eyelid, tarsus

A tarsus, in medical terminology, is a flat surface; most commonly the term refers to the ankle (linking the leg to the flat surface of the foot), but the edge of the eyelid is also a tarsus. Sometimes it will be evident which tarsus is meant, sometimes not; you may have to rely on context to help you.

tarsotomy (TARS-O-tomy) – surgical cutting of a tarsus

tarsophalangeal (TARS-O-PHALANG-eal) – pertaining to the toe bones and the ankle

tarsoclasia (TARS-O-clasia) – surgical fracture of the ankle (to aid correction)

tarsorrhaphy (TARS-O-rrhaphy) – surgical suture of the eyelid, i.e., blepharorrhaphy

metatarsal (*meta*-TARS-al) – pertaining to after the ankle, i.e., pertaining to between the ankle and the toes

Five metatarsal bones extend from the ankle, one to the base of each of the toes. The tarsus of the ankle is actually made up of a group of bones, the talus, calcaneus, navicular, and cuboid, and three cuneiform bones.

2. **TAL—ankle, heel, talus**
   talar (TAL-ar) – pertaining to the talus
   talalgia (TAL-algia) – painful condition of the heel or ankle
   talofibular (TAL-O-FIBUL-ar) – pertaining to the fibula and talus

The talus is the second largest of the bones in the ankle (the largest is the calcaneus); it articulates with the tibia and fibula. While the meaning of talus is quite precise, the meanings "ankle" and "heel" are fairly vague everyday terms. An older term for the talus is astragalus; you may still come across it:

3. **ASTRAGAL—astragalus, talus**
   astragalotibial (ASTRAGAL-O-TIBI-al) – pertaining to the tibia and the talus
   astragalectomy (ASTRAGAL-ectomy) – surgical removal of the talus

4. **CALCANE—heel, calcaneus**
   calcaneal (CALCANE-al) – pertaining to the calcaneus
   calcaneodynia (CALCANE-odynia) – painful condition of the heel
   astragalocalcanean (ASTRAGAL-O-CALCANE-an) – pertaining to the calcaneus and the talus

The smaller bones of the ankle take their names from their shape:

5. **NAVICUL—boat**
   navicular (NAVICUL-ar) – having the character of a boat

6. **CUB—cube**
   cuboid (CUB-oid) – like a cube

7. **CUNE—wedge**
   cuneiform (CUNE-I-form) – like a wedge

So, the navicular bone is boat shaped (it was, at one time, called the scaphoid bone—remember we have already seen the base SCAPH- meaning "boat shaped"), the cuboid bone is cube shaped, and the three cuneiform bones are wedge shaped (we have also seen the base SPHEN- meaning "wedge"). Be careful not to confuse CUB-, "to lie down," with CUB-, "cube."

Compound terms relating to these bones do not always follow the rules that we have been using; cuneocuboid, for example, is used to mean "pertaining to the cuboid and cuneiform bones." You will also come across terms such as cuneonavicular and cuboideonavicular. But, they are generally easy to recognise and figure out.

8. POD—foot
-PUS foot

podiatry (POD-iatry) – medical treatment for the feet

brachypodous (BRACHY-POD-ous) – having feet that are (abnormally) short

podagra (POD-agra) – painful seizure in the foot, i.e., especially the pain in the big toe associated with gout

The form -PUS only occurs at the end of words, so it does not form compound terms of the type we are looking at here. You will find it in nouns such as octopus ("eight feet") and, in medical terminology, in a group of nouns that describe the developmental anomalies associated with legs and/or feet that are fused together—sympus ("together feet" i.e., the feet as well as the legs are fused), apus ("without feet"), monopus ("one foot"), and dipus ("two feet").

We came across the following base previously; remember, only the North American spelling of this base has the alternate meaning "foot":

9. PAED—child
PED—(i) child: (ii) foot

bipedal (BI-PED-al) – pertaining to the feet—two of them

carpopedal (CARP-O-PED-al) – pertaining to the feet and wrists

pedorthics (PED-ORTH-ics) – science of correction for feet, i.e., use of appliances and modified footwear to alleviate foot and lower-limb problems

10. PLANT—sole of the foot

plantar (PLANT-ar) – pertaining to the sole of the foot

plantalgia (PLANT-algia) – painful condition of the sole of the foot

Plantar fasciitis (PLANT-ar FASCI-itis) is an inflammation of the fascia, the thick band of tissue, in the sole of the foot.

We have already met these bases that relate to the toes when we looked at fingers; DIGIT-, DACTYL-, and PHALANG-. Just as there is a special name for the thumb, there is also a special name for the big toe, the hallux (plural halluces):

11. HALLUC—big toe, hallux

hallucal (HALLUC-al) – pertaining to the big toe

subhallucal (*sub*-HALLUC-al) – pertaining to the underneath (surface of the) hallux (bones)

SOME MORE THINGS TO LEARN

Here is our final set of bases to learn:

12. PRUR—itching
PRURIT—itching

prurient (PRUR-I-ent) – pertaining to an itch

pruritic (PRURIT-ic) – pertaining to an itch, pertaining to pruritus

antipruritic (*anti*-PRURIT-ic) – pertaining to (working) against itching

pruritogenic (PRURIT-O-genic) – producing itching

We get the medical terms pruritus (an intense itch) and prurigo (a chronic itchy skin condition) from these bases. The term prurient is not really a medical term; it often has the meaning of "pertaining to a mental itch" for something, i.e., pertaining to a longing or lust for someone or something.

13. PSOR—itching, itchy patches, scaly patches

antipsoric (*anti*-PSOR-ic) – pertaining to (working) against itching

psoriasis (PSOR-iasis) – abnormal condition of scaly patches, i.e., a condition characterized by scaly patches on the skin

psorophthalmia (PSOR-OPHTHALM-ia) – condition of the eye, or eyelid, (characterized by) itching

14. SCAB—itching, scabies
SCABR—itchy patches, scaly patches, rough patches

scabicide (SCAB-I-cide) – substance that kills scabies(-causing mites)

scabious (SCAB-ious) – pertaining to scabies

scabrous (SCABR-ous) – having rough, itchy or scaly patches

scabrid (SCABR-id) – having rough patches

The infection scabies, a highly contagious skin disease, is due to an infestation by certain mites; it is characterized by an itchy rash.

15. CICATR—scar, cicatrix
CICATRIC—scar, cicatrix

cicatrectomy (CICATR-ectomy) – surgical removal of a scar

cicatrization (CICATR-ization) – process of making a scar

cicatricial (CICATRIC-ial) – pertaining to a scar

cicatricotomy (CICATRIC-O-tomy) – surgical cutting of a scar

The medical term for a scar is cicatrix (plural cicatrices). You may occasionally come across the following base meaning "scar," although it is somewhat outdated:

16. UL—scar

uloid (UL-oid) – resembling a scar

ulodermatititis (UL-O-DERMAT-itis) – inflammation of the skin (resulting in the formation of) scars

ulerythema (UL-ERYTH-ema) – condition of reddening (of the skin resulting in the formation of) scars

17. MACUL—spot, macula

macular (MACUL-ar) – pertaining to maculae

maculoerythema (MACUL-O-ERYTH-ema) – condition of reddening (of the skin characterized by) maculae

maculation (MACUL-ation) – process of maculae (formation)

A macula (plural maculae) is a small, discoloured, flat spot on the skin, or an area of tissue that is markedly different from the surrounding tissue.

18. NAEV—mole, birthmark, nevus
NEV—mole, birthmark, nevus

nevoid (NEV-oid) – resembling a nevus

naevomelanoma (NAEV-O-MELAN-oma) – tumor (that appears as a) black mole

nevoxanthoendothelioma (NEV-O-XANTH-O-*endo*-THEL-I-oma) – tumor (arising from an) inside cellular layer (that presents as) a yellow mole, i.e., a yellowish-brown mole that originates from the endothelium

Nevus (or, naevus in British spelling) is the medical term for a mole, or birthmark. As we mentioned previously, melanomas are malignant tumors made up of black or darkly pigmented cells; an endothelioma is generally a benign tumor that originates in the endothelial layer of tissue that lines many vessels in the body, and the heart. Note how, in the term nevoxanthoendothelioma, two bases precede the prefix; we can still use the method, however, that we outlined previously for terms where one base precedes the prefix.

19. PAPUL—papule, pimple

papular (PAPUL-ar) – pertaining to papules

maculopapular (MACUL-O-PAPUL-ar) – pertaining to papules and maculae, i.e., pertaining to a skin condition marked by both papules and maculae

papulosis (PAPUL-osis) – abnormal condition of (numerous) papules

Papules are small, solid, red bumps on the skin.

20. PUSTUL—pustule, pimple

pustulation (PUSTUL-ation) – process (of forming) pustules

papulopustular (PAPUL-O-PUSTUL-ar) – pertaining to (an eruption of both) pustules and papules

pustuliform (PUSTUL-I-form) – having the form of a pustule

Pustules are small bumps on the skin that contain pus.

21. TRAUM—wound, injury, trauma
TRAUMAT—wound, injury, trauma

traumasthenia (TRAUM-asthenia) – weakness (caused through) trauma

traumatopnea (TRAUMAT-O-pnea) – breathing (through) a wound, i.e., air passing through a wound in the chest

atraumatic (*a*-TRAUMAT-ic) – pertaining to without injury, i.e., pertaining to a procedure causing minimal injury

Trauma may be either a physical or mental injury. This is the last of the bases that you have to learn; seems like a fitting one.

Chapter 23

GREEK AND LATIN TERMINOLOGY: SINGULAR AND PLURAL NOUNS

We have now have completed our journey through the body from head to toe. Back in the first chapter, we noted that medical terminology falls basically into three types:

i) Greek and Latin terms that entered the English language in an anglicized form so long ago that we have ceased to think of them as foreign terms,
ii) Greek and Latin terms that entered the English language in their original form, and
iii) compound terms that were systematically devised from Greek and Latin.

We said that the first type should pose little difficulty, at least for English speakers, and we have now looked extensively at the third type, seeing how prefixes, bases and suffixes combine to create thousands of terms. We will spend the remaining chapters looking briefly at the second type.

All of the bases we have looked at are derived from Greek and Latin; they are modified nouns ("things"), adjectives ("describing" words), or verbs ("doing" words), with their endings missing. Many of the nouns, and some of the adjectives, also made their way into medical terminology in their original form. Some we mentioned in passing as we encountered their bases, some we did not. Below is a useful reference list for all the important nouns related to the bases we have learned, along with the chapter numbers in which we met their bases. Almost all of them relate to anatomical features. Some have everyday, non-medical counterparts, some do not and I have listed a definition-type equivalent.

Because these nouns were introduced into medical terminology in their original forms from Greek and Latin, the way that they form their plurals was also incorporated into medical terminology. You need to be able to form and recognize the plurals. A lot of the nouns can be grouped together according to their final letters, and this dictates how the plurals are formed—students of Greek and Latin will recognise these groups as declensions.

NOUNS THAT END IN –A

For nouns that end in –a, replace the –a with –ae. Memorize this rule, and an example that will help you remember it.

cauda	caudae	tail	2
corona	coronae	crownlike structure	2
medulla	medullae	innermost part	4
sclera	sclerae	coating of the eyeball	5
cornea	corneae	transparent layer of the eyeball	5
retina	retinae	light sensitive layer of the eyeball	5
trochlea	trochleae	pulley shaped structure	5
auricula	auriculae	outer ear	6
pinna	pinnae	outer ear, feather, wing	6
fossa	fossae	small depression, hollow	6
concha	conchae	seashell shaped structure	6
cochlea	cochleae	snailshell shaped structure	6
ampulla	ampullae	flask shaped structure	6
ala	alae	wing, wing of a structure	7
papilla	papillae	nipple	8
maxilla	maxillae	upper jaw bone	8
mandibula	mandibulae	lower jaw bone	8
gingiva	gingivae	gum	8
clavicula	claviculae	collar bone	9
scapula	scapulae	shoulder blade	10
ulna	ulnae	bone of the lower arm	10

fascia	fasciae	sheet of connective tissue	10
lamina	laminae	thin plate, layer	10
lamella	lamellae	thin plate, layer	10
crista	cristae	crest, elevated ridge	10
spina	spinae	spine, thorn	10
palma	palmae	palm of the hand	11
vertebra	vertebrae	bone of the spinal column	12
mamma	mammae	breast	12
theca	thecae	cover, sheath	12
bursa	bursae	fluid filled sac	12
trachea	tracheae	windpipe	13
pleura	pleurae	membrane surrounding the lung	13
aorta	aortae	main artery of the body	14
arteria	arteriae	artery	14
vena	venae	vein	14
fenestra	fenestrae	opening	14
plica	plicae	folded structure	17
stria	striae	groove, band, stripe	17
vesica	vesicae	bladder	18
vesicula	vesiculae	small bladder	18
vagina	vaginae	canal from womb to external genitals	19
vulva	vulvae	external female genitals	19
coxa	coxae	hip	21
patella	patellae	kneecap	21
tibia	tibiae	shin bone	21
fibula	fibulae	shin bone	21
macula	maculae	spot	22

THERE IS A SPECIAL GROUP OF NOUNS ENDING IN –A, THE NOUNS THAT END IN –MA

For nouns that end in –ma, replace the –ma with –mata. Memorize this rule, and an example that will help you remember it.

soma	somata	body	2
stoma	stomata	mouth, opening	7
(o)edema	(o)edemata	swelling	10
diaphragma	diaphragmata	diaphragm	10
carcinoma	carcinomata	malignant tumor	20
blastoma	blastomata	malignant tumor	20
sarcoma	sarcomata	malignant tumor	20
trauma	traumata	wound, injury	22

The English language often makes plural nouns by adding an "s." Because it is easy to add an "s" to the Greek and Latin nouns that end in –a or –ma, you will find that plurals such as retinas, corneas, fibulas, carcinomas, for example, are becoming more common and more acceptable. You will find this is especially true in spoken medical language, while written scientific reports do often use the grammatically more correct form.

NOUNS THAT END IN –US

For nouns that end in –us, replace the –us with –i. Memorize this rule, and an example that will help you remember it.

thalamus	thalami	structure within the forebrain	3
gyrus	gyri	fold in the surface of the brain	3
sulcus	sulci	groove in the surface of the brain	3
oculus	oculi	eye	5
canaliculus	canaliculi	small canal, channel	6
ramus	rami	branch of a structure	8

humerus	humeri	upper arm bone	10
radius	radii	bone of the lower arm	10
cubitus	cubiti	elbow, forearm	10
musculus	musculi	muscle	10
carpus	carpi	wrist	11
dactylus	dactyli	finger, toe	11
digitus	digiti	finger, toe	11
arcus	arci	structure shaped like a bow	12
bronchus	bronchi	airway	13
bronchiolus	bronchioli	small airway	13
alveolus	alveoli	cavity	13
thrombus	thrombi	clot	14
embolus	emboli	plug, stopper	14
bacillus	bacilli	rod shaped microorganism	15
coccus	cocci	berry shaped microorganism	15
fungus	fungi	yeast or mold	15
(o)esophagus	(o)esophagi	gullet between throat and stomach	16
umbilicus	umbilici	navel	16
pylorus	pylori	muscular device that opens and closes	16
fundus	fundi	lowest part of an organ	16
villus	villi	hairlike projection	17
glomerulus	glomeruli	ball shaped structure in the body	18
uterus	uteri	womb	19
meniscus	menisci	crescent shaped structure in the body	21
tarsus	tarsi	ankle, eyelid	22
talus	tali	ankle, heel	22
calcaneus	calcanei	heel	22
nevus	nevi	mole, birthmark	22

NOUNS THAT END IN –UM

For nouns that end in –um, replace the –um with –a. Memorize this rule, and an example that will help you remember it.

dorsum	dorsa	back, back part	2
cranium	crania	skull	3
cerebrum	cerebra	principal part of the brain	3
cerebellum	cerebella	area of the hindbrain	3
thelium	thelia	nipple, cellular layer	4
tympanum	tympana	ear drum	6
septum	septa	dividing wall	7
labium	labia	lip, liplike structure	8
frenum	frena	connecting fold limiting movement	8
frenulum	frenula	small connecting fold limiting movement	8
trapezium	trapezia	structure with a trapezium shape	10
brachium	brachia	arm, armlike structure	10
sternum	sterna	breast bone	12
sacrum	sacra	bone at the base of the spine	12
atrium	atria	chamber of the heart	14
serum	sera	watery fluid	14
bacterium	bacteria	microorganism	15
peritoneum	peritonea	membrane in the abdomen	17
omentum	omenta	membrane in the abdomen	17
duodenum	duodena	part of the small intestine	17
c(a)ecum	c(a)eca	blind-ended structure	17
diverticulum	diverticula	small pouch or pocket	17
rectum	recta	lower portion of the intestinal tract	17
ovum	ova	egg	19

perineum	perinea	area between anus and vulva/scrotum	19
scrotum	scrota	pouch that holds the testes	20
ilium	ilia	hip	21
ischium	ischia	lower hip bone	21
acetabulum	acetabula	hip bone socket	21
geniculum	genicula	kneelike structure	21

NOUNS THAT END IN –EX OR -IX

For nouns that end in –ex or –ix, replace the –ex or –ix with –ices. Memorize this rule, and an example that will help you remember it.

cortex	cortices	outer layer	4
helix	helices	spiral	6
cervix	cervices	neck, necklike structure	8
pollex	pollices	thumb	11
apex	apices	tip of a structure	12
radix	radices	root	12
appendix	appendices	structure hanging from another structure	17
calix	calices	cup shaped structure in the body	18
cicatrix	cicatrices	scar	22

Here are two nouns that form their plurals in a similar way: memorize them.

thorax	thoraces	chest	12
hallux	halluces	big toe	22

You may also come across English-type plurals that are becoming more acceptable (for example, cortexes, helixes, and cervixes).

NOUNS THAT END IN –NX

For nouns that end in –nx, replace the –nx with –nges. Memorize this rule, and an example that will help you remember it.

meninx	meninges	membrane	2
pharynx	pharynges	throat	9
larynx	larynges	voice box	9
phalanx	phalanges	finger bone, toe bone	11
salpinx	salpinges	tube	19

Here is a noun that forms its plural in a similar way: memorize it.

coccyx	coccyges	tail bone	12

NOUNS THAT END IN –ON

For nouns that end in –on, replace the –on with –a. Memorize this rule, and an example that will help you remember it.

acromion	acromia	bony projection on the shoulder blade	10
ganglion	ganglia	swelling	12
enteron	entera	intestine	17

THERE ARE EXCEPTIONS TO THESE RULES, AND SOME ODDITIES: USE THESE LISTS FOR REFERENCE, YOU DO NOT NEED TO MEMORIZE THE ENTRIES.

EXCEPTIONS AMONGST THE NOUNS THAT END IN –US

Ones that replace the –us with –era, –ora, or –ura:

latus	latera	side	2
tempus	tempora	temple (on the head)	2
corpus	corpora	body	2
viscus	viscera	internal organ	16
glomus	glomera	ball shaped structure in the body	18
crus	crura	thigh, leg	21

Ones that add –es to the ending (this is an English-type plural that has become acceptable; for some of the terms, you may occasionally see the grammatically correct plural which looks identical to the singular):

meatus	meatuses (or meatus)	passageway, channel	6
sinus	sinuses (or sinus)	hollow cavity	7
virus	viruses	microorganism	15
plexus	plexuses (or plexus)	network of nerves and blood vessels	17
anus	anuses (or anus)	lower opening of the intestinal tract	17
fetus	fetuses (or fetus)	offspring	19

NOUNS THAT END IN –IS

Some of the nouns that end in –is are Greek, and some are Latin; they form their plurals in different ways.

For these nouns that end in –is, replace the –is with –es.

naris	nares	nostril	7
axis	axes	central line, second of the vertebrae	12
sepsis	sepses	presence of toxins in the tissues or blood	15
testis	testes	male reproductive gland	20
pubis	pubes	pubic hair, genitals	21

For these nouns that end in –is, replace the –is with –ides.

iris	irides	colored portion of the eye	5
glottis	glottides	mouth of the windpipe	9
clitoris	clitorides	erectile part of the female genitals	19
epididymis	epididymides	coiled tube on top of the testis	20

COMMON NOUNS THAT DO NOT FALL INTO ANY OF THE CATEGORIES

facies	facies	face, surface	2
psychosis	psychoses	abnormal condition of the mind	3
os	ossa	bone	6
os	ora	mouth	8
caput	capita	head	10
foramen	foramina	opening	12

pons	pontes	bridge of tissue	12
pancreas	pancreata	gland in the abdomen	15
teras	terata	deformed fetus	20
femur	femora	thigh	21
genu	genua	knee	21
didymus	didymoi	testis	20
orchis	orchises	testis	20

Note that any noun that ends in the suffix –osis (neurosis, for example) forms its plural by replacing the –osis with –oses.

This chapter introduced us to quite a number of Greek and Latin nouns in their original form. We had already met their related bases, so most of the meanings should have been fairly familiar. We also learned that we had to obey Greek and Latin grammar to form the plurals of these nouns. We saw that many of the nouns fall nicely into groups that have a simple rule to help us do this.

In whatever area of medicine you go on to study, or in your everyday reading of news topics, or just in regular conversation, you will probably come across some of the terms we have just looked at, both their singular and plural forms.

The terminology we are going to look at in the final couple of chapters, however, is more specialized. Depending on what area of study you continue with, you may, or may not, encounter it. But, at the very least, it is a good idea to be aware of its existence and to have a basic understanding of it. I just want to make a couple of points before we take a deep breath and plunge in.

ANATOMICAL TERMINOLOGY

i) Back in the first chapter, we said that Greek especially was the vehicle for the systematically-developed compound terms, while Latin largely provided the basis for a new anatomical nomenclature. This is the area that we are going to look at, Latin anatomical terminology, so all of the terms from now on are Latin, and they all relate to describing anatomical features.

ii) Many of the terms are not single word terms of the sort we have seen so far; they are phrases, that is groups of two, three, four, maybe even five words, that are the Latin equivalent of, for example, the "descending artery of the knee," or the "elevator muscle of the upper lip."

iii) By the end of the 19th century, the system of Latin anatomical terminology was in a bit of a mess because of regional differences, and there was a move to create an international standard version. This led to the creation of something called the *Nomina Anatomica* ("Anatomical Names"), a standard often referred to by the abbreviation NA. In turn, the NA was replaced at the end of the 20th century by a new standard version, the *Terminologia Anatomica* ("Anatomical Terminology"), or TA. Both NA and TA include English equivalents for the Latin terms (NA is also available in other languages) and you will find many scholarly books and journals that prefer to use English equivalents like "the descending artery of the knee" rather than the Latin forms. But, equally, you will find many scholarly journals and books that prefer the Latin terminology, and you should have some understanding of it, even if it is just enough for you to be able to look up terms effectively in a medical dictionary.

iv) Since the terms come from the Latin language, the rules of Latin grammar have to be applied and obeyed, and a thorough understanding of the material requires a decent grasp of some Latin grammar. Some of you might have this, many of you will not, so we are not going to aim for a thorough understanding, we will be happy with getting a basic understanding, one that you can build on in the future if you need or desire to.

So, deep breath....

Chapter 24

LATIN ANATOMICAL TERMINOLOGY

Suppose you came across a statement like this: "While playing golf, Mr. Smith suffered intense pain in the musculus extensor carpi radialis longus." Or, "Mrs. Jones suffered a blockage in the arteria cervicalis ascendens." What would you make of either of them? You might (now that we have seen them in the previous chapter) recognise musculus and arteria, but as to the other words, radialis and cervicalis look familiar, but the others we don't recognize at all, so what is going on? Both musculus extensor carpi radialis longus and arteria cervicalis ascendens are examples of the Latin anatomical terminology that fills the pages of NA and TA and many scholarly journals (remember, NA is the *Nomina Anatomica*, TA is the *Terminologia Anatomica*); musculus extensor carpi radialis longus is the Latin name of one very specific muscle, while arteria cervicalis ascendens is the Latin name of one very specific artery. We have already seen that musculus and arteria are nouns; the remainder of the terms are made up from other grammatical parts—participles, adjectives, and nouns of a special sort, namely nouns in the genitive case. Let's look at these three grammatical parts.

NOUNS IN THE GENITIVE CASE

What on earth does this mean? We have already seen a number of Greek and Latin nouns ("things") in the previous chapter. All of these nouns are in what is grammatically called the nominative case—this is the form they appear in when they are the subject of a sentence. Well, suppose we want to know the Latin terms that distinguish between the "biceps muscle of the arm" and the "biceps muscle of the thigh." We saw the term biceps in Chapter 10, meaning a "two headed (muscle)," and now we have seen the terms brachium, meaning "arm," and femur, meaning "thigh." But how do we say "of the arm," rather than just "arm," or "of the thigh," rather than just "thigh"? Well, we use the genitive (sometimes called the possessive) case.

In English, we generally indicate the genitive case by adding apostrophe "s" to the end of a word, as in "the day's end," "George's smile," or "the cat's pyjamas." Something similar happens in Latin, but the changes that happen at the end of a word are more variable and we cannot go into the rules that dictate them here. But, so that you can see how these genitive forms are used, here is a list of some common nouns with their genitive forms (and the meaning of the genitive form). Memorize them. When we translate the Latin anatomical terms, we use the English forms:

caput	head	capitis	of the head
cerebellum	cerebellum	cerebelli	of the cerebellum
nasus	nose	nasi	of the nose
labium	lip	labii	of the lip
scapula	shoulder blade	scapulae	of the shoulder blade
brachium	arm	brachii	of the arm
carpus	wrist	carpi	of the wrist
digitus	finger/toe	digiti	of the finger/toe
digiti	fingers/toes	digitorum	of the fingers/toes
femur	thigh	femoris	of the thigh
pes	foot	pedis	of the foot
hallux	big toe	hallucis	of the big toe

With the exception of digiti/digitorum, all of these nouns are in the singular; all plural nouns have their own specific genitive forms, but we will not look at them here.

So to come back to our original question, the "biceps muscle of the arm" is the musculus biceps brachii (often shortened to just biceps brachii), while the "biceps muscle of the thigh" is the musculus biceps femoris (shortened to biceps femoris).

You will also find these genitive forms used in terms such as extensor carpi, "extensor of the wrist," that is a muscle that is responsible for extending or stretching out the wrist. So now we at least know that Mr. Smith's problem was in the extensor muscle of his wrist (musculus extensor carpi), even if radialis longus is still a mystery to us.

We mentioned the types of muscle responsible for certain types of movement back in Chapters 10 and 11. Here they are again:

flexor (FLEX-or)	i.e., muscle that bends a body part
extensor (ex-TENS-or)	i.e., muscle that extends or stretches out a body part
abductor (ab-DUCT-or)	i.e., muscle that draws body part away from the midline
adductor (ad-DUCT-or)	i.e., muscle that draws body part toward the midline
supinator (SUPIN-ator)	i.e., muscle that turns a body part to the supine position
pronator (PRON-ator)	i.e., muscle that turns a body part to the prone position

We can add two other types to this list which we did not discuss:

depressor (de-PRESS-or)	i.e., muscle that lowers a body part
levator (LEV-ator)	i.e., muscle that raises a body part

This base LEV-, which we have not looked at previously, means "raise"; it is not the same as the base LAEV-/LEV- that we met earlier that means "left."

So you may meet terms describing muscles as, for example, flexor carpi, or levator labii. Memorize the anatomical terms for the muscle functional types, and memorize what that anatomical term means. When we translate the Latin anatomical terms, we keep the terms flexor, extensor etc.

You will come across the genitive forms of nouns in many terms, not just ones related to muscles. In the circulatory system, for example, the arteria nasi is an artery of the nose.

ADJECTIVES

We said previously that some adjectives ("describing" words) as well as nouns made their way into medical terminology in their original form. Remember the bases LONG- ("long") and BREV- ("short") and MAGN- ("large, great") from Chapter 11. These bases did not have many compound terms associated with them, but the adjectives from which they are derived, longus, brevis, and magnus, do indeed occur in anatomical terminology; the musculus adductor magnus, for example, is a large adductor muscle. Memorize these three adjectives. When we translate the Latin anatomical terms, we use the English forms:

longus	long
brevis	short
magnus	large, great

We can now also surmise that Mr. Smith's troublesome musculus extensor carpi radialis longus is a long extensor muscle of the wrist. But what about radialis? Well, remember we have seen the base RADI- meaning (amongst other things) "radius of the arm," and we know -alis is a suffix meaning "pertaining to," so radialis is "pertaining to the radius." Mr. Smith's problem is in his long extensor muscle of the wrist on the radial side (i.e., on the same side as his thumb). The suffix -alis is actually an original Latin suffix (-al is the equivalent English form); we have seen it already in temporalis (TEMPOR-alis) and pectoralis (PECTOR-alis).

Here are some Latin adjectives of this type that are common in anatomical terminology. Memorize them (you have already seen their related bases, so it should be easy). When we translate the Latin anatomical terms, we use the English forms (cervical, pectoral etc.):

cervicalis	cervical (i.e., pertaining to the neck or cervix)
pectoralis	pectoral (i.e., pertaining to the chest)
brachialis	brachial (i.e., pertaining to the arm)
radialis	radial (i.e., pertaining to the radius)
tibialis	tibial (i.e., pertaining to the tibia)

Note that some adjectives end in -aris (-ar is the equivalent English form), rather than -alis. Memorize these examples:

scapularis	scapular (i.e., pertaining to the shoulder blade)
ulnaris	ulnar (i.e., pertaining to the ulna)
fibularis	fibular (i.e., pertaining to the fibula)

We have already learned these adjectives:

anterior	i.e., pertaining to the front ("nearer to the front")
posterior	i.e., pertaining to the back ("further to the back")
superior	i.e., pertaining to above ("closer to the higher area")
inferior	i.e., pertaining to below ("closer to the lower area")

Remember, we said that these terms are actually Latin comparative adjectives (the suffix -ior is really a Latin suffix, not an English one), that often mean something like "nearer" and "further," and "higher" and "lower." You will often come across them in relation to things that are found in pairs in the body. When we translate the Latin anatomical terms, we keep the terms anterior, posterior etc.

Here are another two Latin comparative adjectives that often relate to pairs of things. Memorize them. When we translate the Latin anatomical terms, we use the English forms:

major	larger, greater ("larger in size of two similar structures")
minor	smaller ("smaller in size of two similar structures")

PARTICIPLES

Another scary grammatical term, but all we mean here are the sorts of words that end in "ing" in English, such as running, shouting, and making. There is a small group of Latin participles that are used in anatomical terminology; they generally relate to muscles, arteries, veins and nerves, often indicating movement or position. Memorize them, and what the anatomical term means. When we translate the Latin anatomical terms, we use the English forms:

abducens	abducent (i.e., drawing away)
advehens	advehent (i.e., drawing toward)
afferens	afferent (i.e., carrying toward)

efferens	efferent (i.e., carrying away)
ascendens	ascending (i.e., going up)
descendens	descending (i.e., going down)
perforans	perforant (i.e., going through)
recurrens	recurrent (i.e., turning back on itself, or recurring)

So Mrs. Jone's blockage in the arteria cervicalis ascendens occurred in the ascending cervical artery of her neck.

This is all I am going to say about anatomical terminology—hopefully you get the basic idea, and in the final chapter we will look at some examples. I have given you a simplified account here which has largely ignored plural nouns, and has not taken into account the gender of the nouns. In Latin, all nouns have a specific gender (masculine, feminine or neuter), and any adjective or participle that describes a noun has to reflect that gender (as well as whether the noun is singular or plural, and whether the noun is in the nominative or genitive case) by changing its endings. The different endings are numerous (just like we saw for forming plurals); a simple term like longus, for example, can also occur as longa, longum, longi, longae, longorum and longarum and still just mean long in every instance.

On a positive note, if you do need, or desire, to fully master Latin anatomical terminology, it can be reduced to a manageable amount of memorization and the application of a rigid set of rules.

Chapter 25

LATIN ANATOMICAL TERMINOLOGY EXAMPLES

Here are a few examples of anatomical terminology using musculus (muscle), arteria (artery) and vena (vein). Make sure you can understand how we arrived at the English translation. Remember, the terms for the muscle types—flexor, extensor, abductor, adductor, supinator, pronator, levator and depressor—keep their Latin form in the translations, as do the comparative adjectives anterior, posterior, inferior and superior. Think also what the term means, beyond just the translation. What is an abductor muscle of the big toe? What does it do? Where is the brachial muscle located?

1. **musculus brachialis**
   brachial muscle

2. **musculus abductor hallucis**
   abductor muscle of the big toe

3. **musculus adductor magnus**
   large adductor muscle

4. **musculus flexor carpi**
   flexor muscle of the wrist

5. **musculus extensor carpi radialis longus**
   long radial extensor muscle of the wrist

6. **musculus supinator brevis**
   short supinator muscle

7. **musculus pronator pedis**
   pronator muscle of the foot
8. **musculus levator scapulae**
   levator muscle of the shoulder blade
9. **musculus depressor labii**
   depressor muscle of the lip
10. **musculus longus capitis**
    long muscle of the head
11. **musculus pectoralis major**
    greater pectoral muscle
12. **musculus pectoralis minor**
    smaller pectoral muscle
13. **muculus abductor digiti**
    abductor muscle of the finger/toe
14. **musculus extensor digitorum**
    extensor muscle of the fingers/toes
15. **arteria cervicalis ascendens**
    ascending cervical artery
16. **arteria cerebelli inferior anterior**
    anterior inferior artery of the cerebellum
17. **arteria nasi**
    artery of the nose
18. **arteria tibialis posterior**
    posterior tibial artery
19. **arteria recurrens ulnaris**
    recurrent ulnar artery
20. **arteria scapularis descendens**
    descending scapular artery

21. **arteria fibularis perforans**
perforant fibular artery

22. **arteria efferens**
efferent artery

23. **arteria afferens**
afferent artery

24. **arteria cerebelli superior**
superior artery of the cerebellum

25. **venae cerebelli**
veins of the cerebellum

26. **vena cerebri anterior**
anterior vein of the brain

27. **vena advehens**
advehent vein

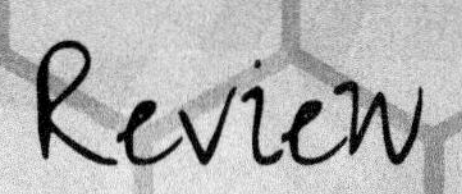

CHAPTERS 21–25

PREFIXES

We did not add any new prefixes to our list.

SUFFIXES

We did not add any new suffixes, or compound suffixes, to our list.

BUILDING UP MEDICAL DEFINITIONS

We saw an example of a term with two bases preceding a prefix:

> nevoxanthoendothelioma (NEV-O-XANTH-O-*endo*-THEL-I-oma) – tumor (arising from an) inside cellular layer (that presents as) a yellow mole, i.e. a yellowish-brown mole that originates from the endothelium

Leave the bases that precede the prefix till last, treat the remaining *prefix*-BASE-suffix in the normal manner (always start with the suffix, then add the prefix, then add in your base) and then add in the other bases last.

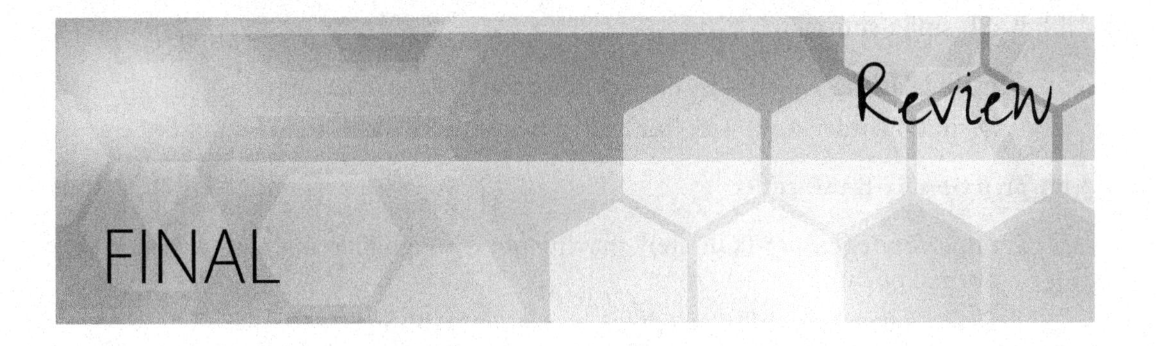

FINAL REVIEW

Congratulations on making it through all the chapters. Do not worry too much if the material on Latin anatomical terminology was a little overwhelming; it is an area that is gradually dropping out of use, with many new textbooks opting to use English equivalents. The compound terms, however, are still firmly entrenched in the medical discipline, and are unlikely to disappear soon. But now you should have no trouble at all distinguishing cardiomalacia, cardiomegaly, and cardiometry; even the dreaded hepatocholangioenterostomy should only cause a brief palpitation.

Here is a final review of the forms of compound terms that we have encountered; remember, there are always rule-breakers and oddities as well. Since combining vowels do not add anything to the sense of the term, we will ignore them here.

These first two forms are at the center of medical terminology; their definition orders do not ever vary.

i) **BASE-suffix**

labiate (LABI-ate) – having lips

Definition order = suffix-BASE

ii) ***prefix*-BASE-suffix**

perignathic (*peri*-GNATH-ic) – pertaining to around the jaw

Definition order = suffix-*prefix*-BASE

For all other forms, we can only talk about generalities; the definition orders and strategies given here are the most common ones, nothing more.

For terms in which there are two suffixes next to each other, or two prefixes next to each other, you generally treat them together, almost as if you are making a single suffix or prefix out of the two:

iii) **BASE-suffix-suffix**

gyroidal (GYR-oid-al) – pertaining to shaped like a coil, i.e., spiral

Definition order = ultimate (last) suffix-penultimate (next to last) suffix-BASE

iv) ***prefix-prefix*-BASE-suffix**

imperforate (*im-per*-FOR-ate) – having not through piercing, i.e., lacking a normal opening

Definition order = suffix-*first prefix-second prefix*-BASE

When there is a base, or bases, preceding a prefix (we would normally expect the prefix to be the first word part), you can often deal with the *prefix*-BASE-suffix part of the term first before addressing the extra base, or bases. If there are several preceding bases, often the technique of moving through bases from right to left can be helpful:

v) **BASE-*prefix*-BASE-suffix**

pupillatonia (PUPILL-*a*-TON-ia) - condition of without tone in the pupil, i.e., the pupil lacks the ability to contract

Treat as regular *prefix*-BASE-suffix, then add the other base

vi) **BASE-BASE-*prefix*-BASE-suffix**

nevoxanthoendothelioma (NEV-O-XANTH-O-*endo*-THEL-I-oma) – tumor (arising from an) inside cellular layer (that presents as) a yellow mole, i.e., a yellowish-brown mole that originates from the endothelium

Treat as regular *prefix*-BASE-suffix, then add the other bases going from right to left

vii) **BASE-BASE-BASE-*prefix*-BASE-suffix**

acrocephalopolysyndactyly (ACR-O-CEPHAL-O-POLY-*syn*-DACTYL-y) – condition of together fingers or toes—many of them, and a head that is (like) the highest point, i.e., condition involving several fused fingers or toes and a head that is peak shaped

Treat as regular *prefix*-BASE-suffix, then add the other bases going from right to left

Sometimes you will come across a term that combines several of these features. Ileoentectropy, for example, has a base preceding two prefixes:

viii) BASE-*prefix-prefix*-BASE-suffix

ileoentectropy (ILE-O-*ent-ec*-TROP-y) – condition of inside outside turning of the ileum, i.e., a turning inside-out of a section of the ileum
Treat as regular *prefix-prefix*-BASE-suffix, then add the other base

Sometimes a term can be broken down into two (or more) simple forms:

ix) BASE-suffix-BASE-suffix

acousticophobia (ACOUS-tic-O-PHOB-ia) – abnormal fear pertaining to sound
Treat as two BASE-suffix forms and then join

Terms with multiple bases are generally the hardest to deal with. Not only do you have to figure out which base, or bases, the suffix and prefix (if there is one) relate to, but you also have to figure out how the bases relate to each other. Other than always starting with the suffix, there are no rules to help; here are some general observations about the terms we have looked at:

x) BASE-BASE-suffix, BASE-BASE-BASE-suffix etc.
***prefix*-BASE-BASE-*suffix*, *prefix*-BASE-BASE-BASE-suffix etc.**

In general, the suffix always relates to the ultimate (last) base:

renotrophic (REN-O-TROPH-ic) – pertaining to the nutrition of the kidneys

It sometimes also relates to the other base(s), in which case we can usually join the bases with "and":

portobilioarterial (PORT-O-BIL-I-O-ARTER-ial) – pertaining to the (hepatic) artery, bile (ducts) and the portal vein

In general, the prefix always relates to the ultimate (last) base:

hyperphotesthesia (*hyper*-PHOT-ESTHE-sia) – condition of more than normal sensation to light

It sometimes also relates to the other base(s), in which case we can usually join the bases with "and":

aglossostomia (*a*-GLOSS-O-STOM-ia) – condition of without mouth and tongue

In general, addressing bases from right to left works well:

> gastroenterohepatic (GASTR-O-ENTER-O-HEPAT-ic) – pertaining to the liver, intestines and stomach

However, you will not always be able to use "and" to join all of the bases:

> hepatocholangioenterostomy (HEPAT-O-CHOLANGI-O-ENTER-O-stomy) – making a surgical opening between the intestines and the bile ducts of the liver

For terms with multiple bases, you really have to think about the most likely common sense solution. Practice will help you a lot, as you will start to see certain patterns emerging with particular combinations of suffixes and bases. Practice will also help you with the other tricky feature of this process, that is getting a feeling for what words need to be added to make accurate, sensible, and usable definitions.

So, practice, practice, practice…

Index

A

B

C

crym (icy cold), 232
crypt (hidden), 29
cryptococcus, 209
cub (cube), 288
cub (to lie down), 123
cubit (elbow, forearm), 123
cubit (to lie down), 123
-culum (small), 94
-culus, -cula, -culum (small), 68, 101, 143, 217
cumb (to lie down), 123
cune (wedge), 288
cusp (cusp), 189
cusp (point, tip), 189
cut/cutane (skin), 32
cyan (blue), 42
cye (pregnancy), 261
cyrt (curved, bent), 160
cyst (bladder, cyst, sac), 49
cyt (cell), 34
-cyte (cell), 32, 61, 147, 221, 276

D

dacry (tears), 52
dactyl (finger, toe), 152
-dactylia, -dactyly (condition of the fingers or toes), 160, 219, 275
de- (down, downward, away from, from, without, out of), 19, 57, 137
de (to bind), 87
dec (ten), 120
dec (tenth), 120
decem (ten), 120
decim (tenth), 120
delph (uterus, womb), 254
delt (delta), 125
dent (tooth), 100
derm/dermat (skin, layer), 17
-desis (surgical fusion, binding), 89, 145, 219, 274
desm (band, ligament), 127
deut (second), 116
deuter (second), 116
dextr (right, right-handed), 13
di (two, twice), 115
dia- (through, apart, in a line), 31
dia-, di- (through, apart, in a line), 38, 57, 138
-dialysis (surgical dissolving, surgical separation, filtration), 89, 145, 219, 274
diaphragm (diaphragm), 133
dich (in two), 115
didym (twin, testis), 266–267
-didymus (twin, conjoined twins), 272, 277
digest (to break apart, to dissolve), 202
digit (finger, toe, digit), 152
dips (thirst), 229–230
dis-, dif-, di- (apart, away from, separation, lack of), 67, 138
dist (away from), 14
diverticul (diverticulum), 239–240
doch (receptacle, duct), 203
dol/dolor (pain), 77
dolich (long), 155
dors (back), 12
drepan (sickle), 195
drepanocyte, 195
duc (to lead, to draw), 129
-duct (duct, channel, tube), 44, 60, 142, 215
duct (to lead, to draw), 129
duoden (duodenum), 237
dur (dura mater), 158
dur (hard), 158
dys- (bad, painful, difficult, abnormal), 19, 57, 138
-dystrophia, -dystrophy (weakness), 174, 219, 275

E

ears
  base(s), 69–80
  prefix(es), 67–68
  suffix(es), 68
ec-, ex- (out, outside), 43, 58, 138
ech (returned sound, repetition), 114
-ectasia, -ectasis (expansion, widening, dilation), 135, 146, 219, 275
ecto- (outside, outer), 10
ecto-, ect- (outside, outer), 38, 58, 138
ectom (to cut out, to cut away), 86
-ectomy (surgical removal, removal), 89, 145, 219, 274
-ectopia, -ectopy (displacement), 135, 146, 219, 275
ede (to swell), 132
-edema (swelling), 275
-(o)edema (swelling), 135, 146, 220
eiso-, eso- (inward), 43, 58, 138
elast (flexible, stretchy), 34

-ellus, -ella, -ellum (small), 101, 143, 217
-ema (condition), 44, 60, 142, 215
embol (insertion, stopper, plug), 196
embry (embryo), 259
embryon (embryo), 259
eme (to vomit), 132
-emesia, -emesis (vomiting), 135, 146, 220
emin (standing out, projecting), 167
-emphraxis (obstruction), 135, 146, 220, 275
en-, el-, em-, er- (in, inward), 19, 58, 138
enanti- (opposite), 67, 138
-ence (state of), 107, 142, 215
encephal (brain), 23
endo- (inside, inner), 10
endo-, end- (inside, inner), 38, 58, 138
endopsychic, 6
enne (nine), 119
-ent (pertaining to), 68, 141, 214
enter (intestine), 235
ento-, ent- (inside, within), 43, 58, 138
enzym (enzyme), 205
epi-, ep- (upon, on the surface), 19, 38, 58, 138
epididym (epididymis), 267
epiplo (epiploon, omentum), 236
episi (vulva), 257
-er (person who (doesà), thing that (doesà)), 68, 142, 215
erythr (red), 40
-esce (to begin, to become), 44, 62, 144, 217
-escent (beginning to be, becoming), 32, 59, 141, 214
-esis (condition, abnormal condition, process), 32, 60, 142, 215
esophag (gullet, esophagus), 223
esthe (to feel, sensation, feeling), 78
-esthesia (condition of sensation), 80, 144, 218, 273
ethm (sieve), 22
-etic (pertaining to), 20, 59, 141, 214
-ety (condition, state, quality), 20, 60, 142, 215
eu- (good, well, normal), 19, 58, 138
eury (wide), 156
ex-, ef-, e- (out, outside, from, without), 67, 138
exo-, ex- (outside, outer, external), 67, 138
-ex or -ix, nouns end in, 299
extern (outside), 14
extra-, extro- (outside of, beyond), 31, 58, 138
eyes
    base(es), 45–53
    prefix(es), 43–44
    suffix(es), 44

F

fac (to make, to cause), 231
faci (face, surface), 14
-facient (making, causing), 277
faec (feces, dung), 241
fasci (band, fascia), 127
febr (fever), 231
fec (feces, dung), 241
feet and toes
    bases, 287–292
female reproductive parts
    bases, 253–264
    suffix, 264
femor (thigh, femur), 281
fenestr (window), 191–192
fer (to bear, to carry, to produce), 35
-ferous (bearing, carrying, producing), 277
ferr (iron), 184
fet (offspring, fetus), 259
fibr (fiber, filament), 171–172
fibrin (fibrin), 172
fibul (fibula), 283–284
-fic (causing, making), 68, 141, 214
-fication (process of producing, process of becoming, process of making), 161, 215
-fici (face, surface), 14
fiss (split, splitting), 24
flav (golden yellow, reddish-yellow), 41
flect (to bend), 128
flex (to bend), 128
foet (offspring, fetus), 259
foll (sac, container), 37
for (to bore, to pierce), 166
foramin (foramen, opening), 166

-form (having the form of, like), 44, 59, 141, 214
foss (ditch, trench, to dig), 71
foss (fossa), 71
fossa ovalis, 2
fratern (brother), 262
fratr (brother), 262
fren (bridle, rein), 96
front (front, forehead), 12
frontal (pertaining to the front), 63
fug (to flee from, to put to flight), 211
-fuge (substance that expels, substance that drives away), 212, 219, 274
fund (fundus), 227
fung (mushroom, fungus), 210
fusc (brown, dark), 41
-fy (to produce, to become, to make), 161, 217

G

galact (milk), 185
gall, 203
gangli (swelling, knot), 171
ganglion, 2
gastr (stomach), 223–224
gemell (twin, paired, born at the same time), 116
gemin (twin, paired, born at the same time), 116
-gen (that which produces), 32, 60, 142, 215
-genesis (production), 80, 147, 221, 277
gen/genit (to produce, to beget), 47
-genic (producing, produced), 80, 147, 221, 277
genicul (geniculum), 282
-genous (producing, produced), 80, 147, 221, 277
ger (to carry, to produce), 201–202
geront (old age), 199
gest (to carry, to produce), 201–202
geus (to taste, sense of taste), 94
-geusia (condition of sense of taste), 105, 144, 218, 273
gingiv (gum), 99
glauc (bluish-gray, silvery-gray), 42
glen (glenoid), 123
glen (socket of a joint), 123
gli (glue), 170
glob (ball, ball shaped), 248
glom (ball shaped), 248
glomer (ball shaped), 248
glomerul (glomerulus), 248–249
gloss (tongue, language), 94
glott
  glottis, mouth of windpipe, 111
  tongue, language, 95, 111
gluc (sweet, sugar), 183
glute (buttocks), 281
glyc (sweet, sugar), 183
gnath (jaw), 98
gon (knee), 282
gon (seed), 254
gonad (gonad), 254
-gram (record), 44, 60, 142, 215
-graph (instrument used to record), 44, 60, 142, 215
graph (to write, to record), 54
-graphy (process of recording), 54, 61, 147, 221, 277
grav (heavy), 157
gravid (pregnant, pregnancy), 157
-gravida (woman who is, or has been, pregnant), 147, 221, 277
greater omentum, 236
gurgit (to flood, to gorge), 230
gust (to taste), 94
guttur (throat), 109
gyn/gynaec/gynec (woman, female), 29
gyr (circle, coil), 25
gyrencephalic (pertaining to the brain), 64
gyroidal (pertaining to shaped like a coil), 64

H

haem (blood), 193
haemat (blood), 193
-haemia, -hemia (condition of the blood), 198, 275
hal (to breathe, breath), 175–176
halluc (big toe, hallux), 289
hands and fingers
  bases, 151–160
  suffixes, 151
haph (touching), 155
hapl (single), 115
hapt (to touch, touching), 155

I

N

nonelastic (pertaining to not flexible), 64
nos (disease, sickness), 78
nose
  base(s), 81–91
  prefix(es), 81
  suffix(es), 81
-nosia (disease), 80, 146, 220, 275
nouns
  falls into no category, 302–303
  in genitive case, 305–307
novem (nine), 119
nutri/nutrit (to nourish, nourishment), 229
-nx, nouns end in, 300
nyct (night), 285

O

ob- (toward, in front of, against), 31, 58, 139
obstetr (obstetrix, midwife), 261–262
obstetr (pregnancy and childbirth), 262
occiput (back of the head), 21
oct (eight), 119
octav (eighth), 119
ocul (eye, sight), 46
odont (tooth), 100
odor (odor, smell), 82
odyn (pain), 77
-odynia (painful condition), 80, 146, 220, 275
oede (to swell), 132
oesophag (gullet, esophagus), 223
-oid (resembling, shaped, like, shaped like), 20, 60, 141, 214
-ol (alcohol (chemistry)), 175, 216
-ole (small), 101, 143, 217
olfact (smell, sense of smell), 81–82
olig (few, scanty), 103
oligomenorrhea, 3
-oma (tumor, mass), 32, 61, 143, 216
oment (membrane, omentum), 236
omphal (navel, umbilicus, umbilical cord), 225
-on, nouns end in, 300
onc (mass, tumor), 270–271
-oncus (tumor, swelling), 272, 275
-one (ketone (chemistry)), 175, 216
oneir (dream), 285
onych (nail), 37
oo (egg), 255
oo (ovum), 255
oophor (ovary), 255–256
ophthalm (eye, sight), 46
-opia (condition of sight), 53, 62, 144, 218, 273
op/ops/opt (eye, sight), 45
-opsia (condition of sight), 53, 62, 144, 218, 274
or (mouth, opening), 94
-or (person who (does…), thing that (does…)), 81, 143, 216
orbit (orbit (of the eye)), 46
orbit (wheel track, circle, ring), 46
orch (testis), 266
orchi (testis), 266
orchid (testis), 266
orect (appetite), 229
orex (appetite), 229
-orium (place for), 20, 61, 143, 216
orth (straight, correct), 159
-ory (having the function of), 68, 141, 214
os (mouth, opening), 94
osche (scrotum), 267
-ose (full of, having the quality of), 32, 60, 141, 214
-ose (sugar (chemistry)), 175, 216
-osis (process of, condition of, abnormal condition of), 20, 61, 143, 216
osm (smell, sense of smell), 82
-osmia (condition of sense of smell), 89, 145, 218, 274
osphres/osphresi (smell, sense of smell), 82
oss/osse (bone), 75
ost (bone), 125–126
oste (bone), 125–126
ot (ear), 70
-ous (pertaining to, like, full of, having), 11, 60, 141, 215
ov (egg), 254–255
ovar (ovary), 255
ovari (ovary), 255
oviduct (oviduct), 255
ovul (ovule), 255
ox
  acute, sharp, pointed, acid-tasting, 180
  oxygen, 180

P

Q

R

S

T

U

V

W

X

Y

Z

CPSIA information can be obtained
at www.ICGtesting.com
Printed in the USA
FSOW04n0501010916
24478FS